AGAINST MEDICAL ADVICE

Addressing Treatment Refusal

Luanne Linnard-Palmer, EdD, RN, CPN
Ellen Christiansen, DNP, RN, FNP-BC, PHNA-BC

Copyright © 2022 by Sigma Theta Tau International Honor Society of Nursing

All rights reserved. This book is protected by copyright. No part of it may be reproduced, stored in a retrieval system, or transmitted in any form or by any means, electronic, mechanical, photocopying, recording, or otherwise, without written permission from the publisher. Any trademarks, service marks, design rights, or similar rights that are mentioned, used, or cited in this book are the property of their respective owners. Their use here does not imply that you may use them for a similar or any other purpose.

This book is not intended to be a substitute for the medical advice of a licensed medical professional. The author and publisher have made every effort to ensure the accuracy of the information contained within at the time of its publication and shall have no liability or responsibility to any person or entity regarding any loss or damage incurred, or alleged to have incurred, directly or indirectly, by the information contained in this book. The author and publisher make no warranties, express or implied, with respect to its content, and no warranties may be created or extended by sales representatives or written sales materials. The author and publisher have no responsibility for the consistency or accuracy of URLs and content of third-party websites referenced in this book.

Sigma Theta Tau International Honor Society of Nursing (Sigma) is a nonprofit organization whose mission is developing nurse leaders anywhere to improve healthcare everywhere. Founded in 1922, Sigma has more than 135,000 active members in over 100 countries and territories. Members include practicing nurses, instructors, researchers, policymakers, entrepreneurs, and others. Sigma's more than 540 chapters are located at more than 700 institutions of higher education throughout Armenia, Australia, Botswana, Brazil, Canada, Colombia, Croatia, England, Eswatini, Ghana, Hong Kong, Ireland, Israel, Italy, Jamaica, Japan, Jordan, Kenya, Lebanon, Malawi, Mexico, the Netherlands, Nigeria, Pakistan, Philippines, Portugal, Puerto Rico, Scotland, Singapore, South Africa, South Korea, Sweden, Taiwan, Tanzania, Thailand, the United States, and Wales. Learn more at www.sigmanursing.org.

Sigma Theta Tau International
550 West North Street
Indianapolis, IN, USA 46202

To request a review copy for course adoption, order additional books, buy in bulk, or purchase for corporate use, contact Sigma Marketplace at 888.654.4968 (US/Canada toll-free), +1.317.687.2256 (International), or solutions@sigmamarketplace.org.

To request author information, or for speaker or other media requests, contact Sigma Marketing at 888.634.7575 (US/Canada toll-free) or +1.317.634.8171 (International).

ISBN: 9781646480500
Epub: 9781646480517
PDF: 9781646480524
Mobi: 9781646480531

Names: Linnard-Palmer, Luanne, author. | Christiansen, Ellen, 1951- author.

| Sigma Theta Tau International, issuing body.

Title: Against medical advice : addressing treatment refusal / Luanne Linnard-Palmer, Ellen Christiansen.

Description: Indianapolis : Sigma Theta Tau International, [2022] |

Includes bibliographical references and index. | Summary: "Refusal, delay or limitation of traditional medical treatments, including vaccines, is an increasing phenomenon. With the desire to apply one's religion, culture, or philosophy, treatment refusals are on the rise. Professionals working in social sciences, medicine, pharmacy, ancillary services as well as nurses in academic environments, professional settings, and advanced practice roles can use this book as a resource to understand the complexity, diversity, and profound impact of pediatric and adult treatment refusals, delays, or limitations. Communication is the central thread throughout the book, as the first step in safety is to assess the individual's or families' beliefs, culture, or philosophical perspectives, understand the impact of these perspectives, share concerns with other healthcare team members, and seek a negotiation or safe outcome for all involved. This book provides the historical background, legal implications, and ethical concerns when individuals or families either limit, refuse, or delay traditional Western medical care based on their religious, cultural, or philosophical beliefs. Findings from recent ethnographic research, clinical guidelines, and latest technology are shared to provide examples of current refusal scenarios and to demonstrate the impact on those involved. This book is written for members of every discipline who are involved with pediatric and adult healthcare including in-patient, critical care, out-patient settings, home care, palliative care, and non-traditional or integral care practices. The center of the struggle is the well-being of the child and adult—no matter what process is utilized to reach treatment goals"-- Provided by publisher.

Identifiers: LCCN 2021041387 (print) | LCCN 2021041388 (ebook) | ISBN 9781646480500 (paperback) | ISBN 9781646480517 (epub) | ISBN 9781646480524 (pdf) | ISBN 9781646480531 (mobi)

Subjects: MESH: Treatment Refusal | Patient Compliance | Parental Consent | Cultural Competency

Classification: LCC R733 (print) | LCC R733 (ebook) | NLM W 85 | DDC 615.5--dc23

LC record available at https://lccn.loc.gov/2021041387

LC ebook record available at https://lccn.loc.gov/2021041388

First Printing, 2021

Publisher: Dustin Sullivan
Acquisitions Editor: Emily Hatch
Development Editor: Meaghan O'Keeffe
Cover Designer: Becky Batchelor
Interior Design/Page Layout: Becky Batchelor
Indexer: Larry Sweazy

Managing Editor: Carla Hall
Publications Specialist: Todd Lothery
Project Editor: Carla Hall
Copy Editor: Todd Lothery
Proofreader: Erin Geile

FREE BOOK RESOURCES

To download a printable tips page for dealing with against medical advice situations, a sample chapter, and other book-related materials, visit the *Against Medical Advice* Sigma Repository page via the link or QR code below.

http://hdl.handle.net/10755/21755

ACKNOWLEDGMENTS

From Dr. Luanne Linnard-Palmer:

Thank you, my precious family:
Evan, you are so wonderful and calm.
Logan, you couldn't be more inquisitive, wiser, or understanding.
Christina, your energy is inspiring and transformational.
Mom, you are always there to support, love, and provide professional guidance.
My family melts my heart.
Loren, Judith, Dean, Heather, Doug, Jessica, and Danielle,
Thank you for your faith in me.
Dad, I miss you every minute of every day. Life is not the same without you.
Love and blessings to you in heaven.

From Dr. Ellen Christiansen:

Many heartfelt thanks to Patty Bradford, who cared for me as a patient before I knew what a nurse practitioner was. (I assumed she was a physician.) Ours has been one of my most enduring and meaningful friendships.

Many thanks to Jane, Marty, Diane, Dale, Diney, Carrie, and Mary for leading by example. You are all such amazing clinicians!

DISCLAIMER

The authors' intent for this book is to accurately describe the perspectives and beliefs of various religious, cultural, and philosophical perspectives and groups on medical care and vaccines, as well as to provide reports from lawyers, researchers, and academics—all without malice, judgment, or persecution. The information presented in this book came directly from current or past literature, medical internet sources, or direct quotes from personal communications received by the authors. The perspectives shared by sources summarized for this book do not necessarily represent the views or religious beliefs of the authors. The authors did not intend to disclose personal perspectives on the critical topics of adult, parent, or child refusal, delay, or limitation of medical treatment or vaccines for religious, cultural, or philosophical beliefs, doctrines, or perspectives. Every attempt has been made to ensure the accuracy of the content of this book; however, any inaccurate report of religious beliefs, facts, quotes, or historical events is accidental and regrettable.

This book was not intended to pass judgment on the existence of divine, supernatural, or spiritual realms. The authors do not wish or intend to pass judgment on religious decisions or beliefs of any kind. Rather, the intent of the book is to offer guidance and a foundation for critical analysis and discussions for those involved with treatment/vaccine refusal situations.

ABOUT THE AUTHORS

Luanne Linnard-Palmer, EdD, RN, CPN, is a Professor of Nursing at Dominican University of California in San Rafael, California, and a Pediatric Educational Consultant and Pediatric Clinical Nurse at Sutter Health's California Pacific Medical Center in San Francisco. She received her undergraduate nursing degree from Humboldt State University and began clinical practice in oncology. She received her master's degree from the University of San Francisco School of Nursing and her EdD at the University of San Francisco School of Education in the Department of Curriculum Development and Instructional Design. She has taught in several nursing programs in the San Francisco Bay Area and now holds tenure at Dominican University of California. She studied the topic of parental refusal of traditional medical care during her post-doctoral studies at the University of California in the Department of Family Health Care Nursing, San Francisco, under the direction of Dr. Susan Kools. She completed two ethnographic studies during her post-doctoral program (2000–2003) and is writing this book as a cumulative project that represents personal clinical experiences as a pediatric oncology/hematology nurse, a nursing instructor who takes students to large urban hospitals rich with diverse populations, and an ethnoscience researcher.

Her hope for this book is that she can influence healthcare professionals to treat families with the utmost respect; to encourage careful listening; to contemplate the legitimacy of parents' opinions, wishes, and beliefs; and to ensure that all children will receive necessary care to prevent human suffering, disease, illness, disability, or death.

She also hopes that the reader will come away with a strong sense of legal duty and will uphold the laws that have been carefully constructed to protect our nation's children. The book has not been written to express the personal opinions of this author but rather to educate pediatric healthcare professionals on the entire subject of parental refusal of medical care based on religious or cultural beliefs.

There is no way around the topic in influential treatment decisions made by parents. A career in pediatric healthcare means encountering these families for whom rich cultural preferences or deeply held religious convictions influence medical treatment decisions. To be sure, the larger, more chaotic urban hospitals, especially those that are teaching and/or research hospitals, will serve a larger population of diverse families. Nevertheless, all healthcare professionals should be prepared to handle these delicate and highly charged human interactions.

She hopes you find this book helpful in your professional practice and an enjoyable reading experience.

Ellen Christiansen, DNP, RN, FNP-BC, PHNA-BC, is an Associate Professor of Nursing at Dominican University of California, where she teaches Community and Public Health Nursing to first semester senior nursing students. She is also responsible for securing interesting educational community-based placements where her students can learn about population health and make a real contribution to the health of the community. Christiansen received her baccalaureate degree in nursing from Dominican University of California. During undergraduate nursing school, she began to understand the importance of the social determinants of health, and she became passionate about social justice. She also realized that she loved working with a multicultural, underserved patient population, and she preferred doing it in a community-based setting. Accordingly, she enrolled in Samuel Merritt University and obtained her master's in nursing as a family nurse practitioner. She spent the next several years working in three rural, federally qualified community health centers on the coast of Northern California. Eventually, she attended Sonoma State University for a certification in Rural Community Clinic Management, and she became the Director of Operations for the three community clinics. Finally, having worked a total of 17 years for the community

ABOUT THE AUTHORS

health centers, Christiansen's interest turned to nursing education, and she returned to Samuel Merritt University, where she obtained a DNP degree. Afterward, she taught part time for Samuel Merritt University but was soon hired for a full-time tenure track position at Dominican University of California, where she still teaches today as a tenured Associate Professor.

About six years ago, Christiansen began taking her community health nursing students out to the same rural area where she had worked as a family nurse practitioner. There (among other things) the students performed home visits to older adults attempting to safely age in place in their homes, remaining in the very beautiful but isolated rural area they had lived in for many years, trying to avoid institutionalization in skilled nursing facilities. Often, the nursing students could see very clearly what the older adults needed to do to maximize their health and well-being, yet the older adults frequently failed and/or refused to do it. This sparked Christiansen's interest in investigating the issues around patients who refuse, delay, or modify their treatment for religious, philosophical, cultural, or other reasons. Christiansen looks forward to sharing what she has discovered, and she hopes the information will assist other nurses in caring for their patients more effectively—especially when those patients are contemplating making a choice against medical advice.

CONTENTS

About the Authors vii
Foreword xvii
Introduction xix

1 WHEN MEDICAL TREATMENT AND PATIENT NEEDS CLASH 1
    Children and Their Families 3
    Nineteen Case Examples of Refusal Scenarios 5

2 OVERVIEW AND REASONS FOR TREATMENT REFUSALS 21
    Factors Associated With Treatment Refusals 22
    Additional Reasons for Treatment Refusal. 25

3 CHILDHOOD VACCINES, HESITANCY, AND REFUSALS 31
    Types of Vaccines. 32
    Summary of Parental Concerns to Vaccines and Suggested Responses 35
    Vaccine Hesitancy 41
    Laws and Exemptions Related to Childhood Vaccines. 42

4 PEDIATRIC HEALTHCARE, ETHICS, AND CHILDREN'S RIGHTS. 47
    Children's Rights 48
    Ethics. 53

5 **LEGAL IMPLICATIONS AND CONSENT: INFORMED CONSENT, ASSENT, AND PARENTAL PERMISSION** 59
  Informed Consent. 60
  Assent 61
  Parental Permission 62

6 **LEGAL PERSPECTIVES OF TREATMENT REFUSAL: REFUSAL DEFINED** 65
  Routes of Legal Actions. 67
  Historical Perspectives of Treatment Refusal..... 71

7 **IN THE NAME OF RELIGION: HISTORICAL INFLUENCES TO LEGAL EXEMPTIONS** 75
  Historical Influences. 77
  Clergy Responsibility and the Law. 81
  Legal Exemptions to Specific Types of Healthcare/Treatments 83

8 **ADULT MEDICAL TREATMENT REFUSALS, LIMITATIONS, AND DELAYS** 87
  Medication Nonadherence 89
  Communication Techniques for Adult Refusals, Limitations, and Delays. 90
  Global Perspectives on Health, Illness, and Treatment. 96
  Individual Worldview and Its Impact on Healthcare Decisions 97

Avoidant Health-Seeking Behaviors in the Black
Community 98
Belief in Alternative Therapies 102
Adult Vaccine Refusal and Hesitancy 105
Distrust of Vaccines on the Global Level. 108

9 **OVERVIEW OF RELIGIOUS DOCTRINES** **111**

Churches With Frameworks Supporting Refusal
of Medical Treatment, Limitation, or Delay. 112
Types of Prayer and Religiosity That Influence
Children's Healthcare Decisions 115
Clerical Interpretations 119
Specific Religious Doctrines Defined 121

10 **THE IMPORTANCE OF CULTURAL
COMPETENCE** **145**

Theoretical Influences: Decision-Making Models. . . 149
Decision-Making Models 151
Emotional Reactions and Moral Distress in
Refusal Scenarios. 154

11 **PROFESSIONAL GROUPS' REACTIONS TO
TREATMENT REFUSAL: NURSING, MEDICINE,
RESEARCHERS, AND JOURNALISTS** **161**

Nursing 162
Physicians. 163
Professional Journalists: Current and Historical
Perspectives 165

12 OVERVIEW OF PROFESSIONAL INTERVENTIONS: POWER DISTANCE, NEGOTIATION, AND SAFETY 171

Ethnographic Research in Treatment Refusal Cases. 173
Conclusion 184

A REASONS FOR PARENTAL DECISIONS TO REFUSE MEDICAL TREATMENT 187

B GUIDELINES FOR STAFF FACING PARENTAL REFUSAL OF PEDIATRIC VACCINES OR MEDICAL TREATMENTS 191

C GUIDELINES FOR STAFF FACING ADULT REFUSAL OF MEDICAL TREATMENTS. 195

D LOSS OF PARENTAL GUARDIANSHIP: COURT OVERRIDING OF A PARENT'S RIGHT TO REFUSE MEDICAL TREATMENT 197

What Is Guardianship? 197
Five Reasons for Courts to Override a Patient's Right to Refuse Medical Treatment 200

E COMMON CONCERNS ABOUT VACCINE ADMINISTRATION 203

F PANDEMICS AND TRUST IN RAPID VACCINE CREATION, DISTRIBUTION, AND MANDATES. . . 207

CONTENTS

G BEST INTEREST AND THE LAW: SHOULD STATE STATUTES ON CHILD ABUSE BE MODIFIED? ... 209

H SPIRITUAL ABUSE DEFINED ... 211

I RESOURCES FOR MORE INFORMATION ... 213
    General Resources ... 213
    Websites on Treatment Refusal ... 214
    Useful Resources to Assist in the Management of Patients Who Refuse Blood Transfusions ... 214
    Resources Available for Children, Parents, and Adults Regarding Vaccines ... 215

REFERENCES ... 219

INDEX ... 237

FOREWORD

The intersection between science and decisions regarding treatment options remains complex and challenging for healthcare professionals and families. Medical, legal, social, cultural, and religious perspectives influence critical choices impacting the health and welfare of both adults and children. Understanding reasons for refusing, limiting, or delaying important healthcare treatment decisions can be valuable for all involved. The purpose of this book is to provide a legal, social, cultural, and ethical context in which to place healthcare decisions in significant clinical context. As noted by the authors, the book emphasizes that healthcare professionals need to recognize, acknowledge, and negotiate with members of different religious and cultural groups to promote excellent care delivery.

The authors initially begin their investigation of treatment refusal through a series of seven questions. The questions address the history of child and parental rights, the development of laws affording professionals rights to administer treatments, the ethical principles associated with mandated treatments, the identification of religious groups, and the cultural, religious, and philosophical beliefs influencing delay or refusal of Western traditional healthcare. Questions about the effects of treatment refusal affecting children, families, and clinicians, and the exploration of individual state laws regarding immunization prior to public school entry, also form questions for further inquiry. This approach provides a helpful framework for recognizing issues associated with decisions to defer or refuse a number of medically recommended or required interventions.

The book provides the reader with a comprehensive guide to a number of cultural and religious factors associated with treatment refusals. Chapters explores pediatric healthcare ethics, legal perspectives in pediatric and adult treatment refusal, religious and cultural factors, global perspectives on treatment refusal, and information on ethnographic inquiry and perspectives on power distance.

AGAINST MEDICAL ADVICE

Staff guidelines for parental refusal of vaccinations or medical treatments, information about common concerns regarding vaccine administration hesitancy and refusal, and identification of religious groups influential in healthcare treatment decisions are integrated in the book.

Of critical relevance are the updates focused on the COVID-19 pandemic–related resistance to vaccinations and quarantine, as well as lack of trust in rapid vaccine creation, mandates, and distribution. This information is especially beneficial to healthcare providers facing difficult decisions during the current COVID-19 pandemic.

From the historical overview of treatment refusals to information relevant to the current COVID-19 pandemic, the authors of this book explore significant legal, ethical, social, religious, and cultural issues related to the important topic of healthcare decision-making. This book provides a careful and thoughtful approach to a topic of great importance to healthcare professionals and families.

–Dr. Andrea Boyle, RN
Chair and Associate Dean, Department of Nursing
School of Health and Natural Sciences
Dominican University of California

INTRODUCTION

The term *Against Medical Advice* (AMA), also known as *Discharged Against Medical Advice* (DAMA) or *Leaving Against Medical Advice* (LAMA), was coined in approximately 1950 and means to leave a healthcare institution or the care of a physician against the advice of one's doctor (Godfrey, 2017). If patients are deemed competent in their decision-making, then they are entitled to decline recommended medical treatment and take responsibility for their clinical outcomes. They must be told of the risks, benefits, and consequences of their decision and subsequent action. According to recent research, the highest risk factors for individuals leaving AMA are male gender, substance abuse disorder, and low socioeconomic status (Alfandre, 2013), as well as Black race, lack of health insurance, homelessness, and those with psychiatric disorders or HIV/AIDS (Godfrey, 2017). AMA status is increasing exponentially, with approximately 500,000 cases occurring per year (Alfandre & Schumann, 2013). One study demonstrated that between 1997 and 2011, there was a 41% increase in the incidence (Pfuntner et al., 2013). As stated by Alfandre and Schumann (2013), "The risks to these patients are significant. Compared with patients discharged conventionally, readmission rates for patients discharged AMA are 20% to 40% higher, and their adjusted relative risk of 30-day mortality may be 10% higher" (p. 2393). Many wonder if medical insurance will pay for a hospitalization when one leaves AMA. Little research could be found that confirms the trend in this question. One article by Huntsbery-Lett (2020) describes a study conducted at the University of Chicago Medical Center where data showed that out of 50,000 medical records with 453 patients who left AMA, no patients were denied medical insurance coverage for the care they received. For this text, the focus is on refusing medically prescribed treatments or routine health maintenance and vaccines against the advice and direction of a healthcare professional. Three very important questions have been posed concerning AMA:

1. If patients do not have sufficient information or understanding to make informed decisions, are they in fact leaving AMA?

2. Shouldn't health literacy be a consideration in AMA discharges? (Godfrey, 2017)

3. Do patients who refuse medical treatment understand that there is a much higher risk for complications and poor outcomes?

The literature has disclosed a variety of perspectives on treatment refusal scenarios which can occur because of people's cultural, philosophical, or religious beliefs. These treatment refusals can be particularly challenging for healthcare providers to deal with when parents wish to withhold medical treatment from a child based on the family's closely-held religious beliefs. See the quotes below for various viewpoints from the healthcare community.

> We commonly excuse parents, legally and morally, for inflicting upon their children what most people would regard as harm when the parents act on the basis of religious belief. While states have prosecuted some parents for causing their children to die by failing to obtain necessary medical care, even though the parents had sincere religious objections to medical care, these few cases represent only the most extreme situations and mask a *quite widespread but generally overlooked phenomenon.* (Dwyer, 1996, p. 1)

> The battle between health professionals' desire to treat child illness while applying all known technology and the religious doctrines of faithful parents has become *a legal war.* (Anonymous, 2001)

> There has been some scientific evidence that religious beliefs and prayer have psychological benefits that may in fact contribute to a person's illness recovery. Churches, on the other hand, have published testimonials that functional and organic diseases can be healed by what is called divine power, yet this has not been scientifically confirmed with valid measurement. (Asser & Swan, 1998, para. 2)

INTRODUCTION

The emphasis of this book is on the imminent need for healthcare professionals to acknowledge the presence of these individuals and groups in our current society and plan for interactions that promote education and negotiation for the best possible care for children and adults.

The prevalence of religious groups and cultural groups emphasizing prayer or cultural behaviors over traditional Western medical care is unknown, but reports of the phenomenon are growing in the US. According to the website www.religioustolerance.org, J. Gordon Melton, Director of the Institute for the Study of American Religion, described to ABC News (2002) that more people who turn to prayer rather than medical care for their children are getting charged with crimes. Melton reported that those who have criminal charges are often members of charismatic Christian groups who base their decisions on certain scriptures—especially from Acts and Paul's epistles.

It is the intent of this book to cover historical aspects of many religious, cultural, and philosophically minded groups without comparing their religious or spiritual frameworks, as each is separate and unique. Frameworks shared in this book are presented as accurately as possible using a wide variety of sources.

The value of love and concern for individuals and their children or a group's members and children is not in question; rather, this book aims to explain all aspects of the phenomena of refusal, delay, or limitation of treatment, including *why*. It is often through love that one applies religious or cultural beliefs or a closely held philosophical perspective, so the concern for and commitment to the child or adult is recognized. The concern is the outcome of the application of these deeply held beliefs on the ultimate well-being of the person and the person's health state.

EIGHT QUESTIONS THAT GUIDED THE RESEARCH

Eight broad questions guided the investigation of literature, in-depth interviews, and ethnographic research studies that led to the writing of this book. These questions are shared to give clarity on how the phenomenon of pediatric and adult treatment refusal was first studied.

1. What are the historical events that have taken place over the last 100 years that have moved the perspective of a child from being "property without rights" to having rights that supersede the constitutional rights of parents?

2. How have the laws developed that provide healthcare professionals the opportunity to seek and secure legally mandated temporary guardianship to administer lifesaving medical treatment or treatments to alleviate human suffering against the religious or cultural doctrines of families?

3. What states have enacted laws requiring childhood vaccines prior to entering public school, and how have those concerned about childhood vaccines reacted to these state laws?

4. What are the ethical principles at stake surrounding mandated treatment with or without the loss of guardianship? What are the ethical principles surrounding parents' authority to make decisions for their children? What ethical principles are related to decision-making of adults and their desire to refuse, limit, or delay needed medical treatment?

5. What are the primary examples of religious, cultural, and philosophical beliefs whose doctrines influence alternative, limited, delayed, or refused healthcare treatment modalities? What are exemplary illustrations of situations of refusal for

each? How do adult refusals versus child/family refusals differ?

6. How does the situation of refusal and subsequent mandated treatment affect the child, family, individual, and community of health professionals? Is moral distress a frequently encountered outcome or a rare endpoint of extreme cases?

7. Who are these religious groups? Where are they located? How influential are they, and what exactly do they believe? Are religious doctrines and church membership changing? Who are the cultural groups whose norms influence parental healthcare decisions, and what are their beliefs? Which community-based organizations are currently providing information and guidelines for vaccine refusal?

8. How do healthcare professionals prepare for treatment refusal discussions, whether they are as life-threatening as surgeries, transfusions, or chemotherapy or less significant yet also potentially lifesaving as refusing vaccines? (Refusing a vaccine for COVID-19 is an example of the significance of vaccine refusal.)

Professionals working in the social sciences, medicine, pharmacy, and ancillary services—as well as nurses in academic environments, professional settings, and advanced practice roles—can use this book as a resource to understand the complexity, diversity, and profound impact of pediatric and adult treatment refusals, delays, and limitations.

Communication is the central thread throughout this book, as the first step in safety is to assess an individual's or family's beliefs and cultural or philosophical perspectives and to understand the impact of these perspectives, share concerns with other healthcare team members, and seek a negotiation or safe outcome for all involved.

CHAPTER 1

WHEN MEDICAL TREATMENT AND PATIENT NEEDS CLASH

As immigration rates continue to grow, urban populations explode, vaccine technology advances, and church membership increases, healthcare team members will more frequently encounter a wide array of cultural, religious, and philosophical perspectives toward medical treatments and vaccines. Some of these situations will go smoothly, and some will not. Medical treatment refusal cases have the potential to result in child and adult injuries and deaths, making it imperative that every member of the healthcare team be knowledgeable about how to react to treatment refusals and how to communicate and work with family, clergy, and organized groups to create an environment for optimal outcomes.

Nurses, physicians, and related healthcare professionals are in a unique position to offer support to families who are experiencing the critical dilemma of wanting prayer in lieu of medical care, or wishing to limit medical care based on cultural, religious, or philosophical doctrines. Although the healthcare professionals involved may not agree with the application of parental cultural or religious beliefs on medical decision-making and may proceed with securing state guardianship and mandated treatment for children involved, families and individuals deserve respect and a voice. They deserve the opportunity to explain their beliefs and preferences, alone or in the presence of their clergy or elders, when time is not restricted by the critical status of the child's or adult's condition. They also deserve the opportunity to apply religious or cultural practices when safe and appropriate in the healthcare setting. Healthcare professionals can minimize the stress, fear, anxiety, and possible anger of family members by demonstrating an understanding of diverse beliefs and allowing time, whenever safe and possible, for each family member to disclose their concerns, belief systems, and cultural practices.

Healthcare professionals who encounter families of diverse cultural and religious backgrounds must be knowledgeable about legal and ethical principles, as well as the basic foundations of various religious doctrines. Healthcare professionals can be better prepared to participate in treatment decisions if they are well-versed in a variety of literature (and on how to retrieve the literature) and are aware of the many viable perspectives on treatment refusal.

This book discusses the historical background, legal implications, and ethical concerns when individuals or families limit, delay, or refuse conventional (also known as allopathic) Western medical care based on their religious, cultural, or philosophical beliefs. Findings from recent ethnographic research, clinical guidelines, and the latest technology are shared to provide examples of current refusal scenarios and to demonstrate the impact on those involved. Numerous references, websites, and current literature are offered to disclose the impact of this highly charged dilemma, as well as examples of actual refusal situations and their outcomes. Practice guidelines are presented with the focus on assessment, communication, and resolution for the administration of safe and legal interdisciplinary care during refusal situations.

CHILDREN AND THEIR FAMILIES

When all is well, healthcare professionals carry out their practice administering care deemed appropriate for a select child or adult who is experiencing an identified disease or disorder or who requires preventative treatments such as well-child/adult visits and vaccines. When an individual refuses recommended treatment or sets limitations on which treatments or diagnostic exams will be allowed, the harmony changes, and the situation can become problematic. Everyone now becomes concerned, yet few may know exactly what to do and how to progress. In these delicate situations, the ultimate concern is not who has the final say but rather the physical and emotional well-being of the child and the education and support of the adult.

American culture has placed great value on the autonomy of a parent's decisions for their child. These decisions include education, discipline, socialization, safety, and recreation. When it comes to medical decisions, our culture trusts that a parent will provide one of the most basic of human needs: competent healthcare. Although there are many reasons for parental refusal of a child's medical care, the application of religious and cultural beliefs can be most profoundly influential. For adults, our culture honors autonomy and self-direction in decision-making. The focus of this book is on the various religious doctrines and cultural beliefs whose ultimate practice influences adults' and parents' views and opinions on the application of healthcare, and on the legal, moral, and ethical processes that occur simultaneously.

AGAINST MEDICAL ADVICE

Upon being asked, most healthcare professionals report having encountered at least one if not many refusal situations. Many say this ethical dilemma leaves a lasting mark on their memory, or sometimes their career. The refusal scenarios may go smoothly, but other times, even with a multidisciplinary approach, the refusal scenario is highly charged. This situation becomes complex when a parent loses guardianship of a child to the state for the time required to apply lifesaving treatments, or when an adult suffers disability or death. For families, mandated treatment is avoided whenever possible to keep relations smooth and the family on board for subsequent healthcare needs.

Many healthcare professionals report feeling ill-prepared to negotiate with the family during treatment refusals, especially vaccine refusals, as many report having minimal knowledge about the legal requirements or a lack of knowledge about the religious doctrines or cultural beliefs that families hold dear. It is imperative that pediatric and adult healthcare professionals have access to resource materials to guide them through treatment refusal scenarios (see Appendix I for a list of resources). Knowing the legal influences, knowing their professional roles and responsibilities, and knowing about various religions and cultures whose doctrines influence healthcare decisions—*and knowing how to best communicate*—is crucial. It is most distressing for the family if their treatment wishes cannot be honored. It is also very difficult for the healthcare professionals involved to have to give time-consuming and often morally distressing energy toward negotiations that are at times futile. It is quite apparent, through personal experiences as well as disclosures via interviews, that most people want to avoid "battles" or highly charged disagreements over treatment decisions altogether. But avoiding these battles is often not easy to do.

This book aims to clarify aspects of conventional (allopathic) Western medical treatment refusal (or limitation) and to provide avenues for additional resources. It is written for members of every discipline who are involved with pediatric and adult healthcare, including inpatient, critical care, outpatient settings, home care, palliative care,

1 WHEN MEDICAL TREATMENT AND PATIENT NEEDS CLASH

and nontraditional or integral care practices. Again, the center of the struggle is the well-being of the child or adult, no matter what process is utilized to reach treatment goals.

NINETEEN CASE EXAMPLES OF REFUSAL SCENARIOS

To understand the magnitude and impact of medical treatment limitation, delay, or refusal, it is important to first understand the situations that bring the adult or child into the healthcare arena. The following 19 cases provide brief examples of medical treatment refusal scenarios. Some of the examples are from the authors' ethnographic investigations and interviews, some are from recent media or internet sources, and others are narratives shared by concerned colleagues. The selected examples are stories, or narrations, shared by others through individual eyes and perceptions. Without a doubt, the following examples present a variety of perceptions depending on personal views, beliefs, life experiences, and memories of those involved.

CASE 1: REFUSING TRANSFUSIONS

Upon arriving at work on a Saturday morning in October, an experienced registered nurse who specialized in pediatric hematology and oncology care approached the nursing station at a large urban pediatric hospital to find an unusually large number of doctors, interns, residents, nurses, and family members standing in the hallway near the nurse's station. She received report and was informed that a 4-year-old boy, very ill with sickle cell anemia, would be her patient that day. The child's bloodwork demonstrated very severe anemia (a hemoglobin of 4.9 gm/dL), and he required an emergent blood transfusion. The family was refusing transfusion therapy as they were devout Jehovah's Witnesses. The pediatrician in charge of the care of the child raised his voice slightly and informed the family and clergy present that there was no more time to negotiate alternatives as the child was tachycardic, listless, and could experience serious consequences of delayed therapy. The pediatrician called the hospital social services department, hospital administration, and the county court representatives. He was able to secure temporary legal guardianship for mandated treatment for the time period required to administer the lifesaving blood transfusion therapy.

The parents were distraught but cooperated with the procedures. As the morning unfolded, the family shared with the nurse their beliefs about the possible consequences of the blood transfusion on the child's soul, his future relationship with God, and his chances of arriving safely in heaven (Anonymous, personal communication, October 15, 2004).

CASE 2: FAITH AND DISEASE

A 9-year-old girl was brought to a large urban pediatric hospital via helicopter after a neighbor notified the county authorities of her medical condition. This young girl had stepped on a nail while visiting a national park with her family and had not been immunized for tetanus. She subsequently developed severe osteomyelitis from the puncture site in her foot up to her hip with severe swelling, redness, pain, and loss of function. When the neighbor of the family noticed the condition of the child, she was being administered prayer from faithful Christian Science practitioners in the home. The child's medical condition warranted six weeks of intensive antibiotic therapy while hospitalized. Unable to obtain the parents' written consent, the court agreed to grant temporary legal guardianship for the time period needed to treat the infection via a peripherally inserted central venous catheter. The family was present at the bedside and provided loving support to the child during her hospitalization (Anonymous, personal communication, November 2003).

1 WHEN MEDICAL TREATMENT AND PATIENT NEEDS CLASH

CASE 3: NEED FOR CULTURAL CARE

A 14-year-old Muslim child was recovering from a first-degree burn to the elbow from spilling boiling hot cooking oil while in her family's kitchen. The child had had extensive surgical reconstruction, and her arm was slowly healing with a skin graft placed over the surgical site. While her extended family was visiting her at the bedside in a large Midwestern pediatric burn center, the medical team conducted bedside morning rounds to assess the child and her burn site. While talking among the team in the child's hospital room, the surgeon was overheard by the family stating that the pig's skin graft was adhering well and leading to successful lower tissue repair. The family became very distraught that they had not been informed of the child's reception of pig tissue and demanded that the graft be removed. The child went back to surgery, the graft was removed, and the child experienced almost complete loss of function of her upper extremity. Nevertheless, the family was appeased and satisfied that their cultural requirements were upheld (Anonymous, personal communication, October 2003).

CASE 4: HANDS-ON PRAYER

A teenage patient of an outpatient oncology unit had just been diagnosed with a rapid-growing lymphoma located on her neck. The family, clearly distraught, requested to have three to five days of comprehensive prayer conducted among their fellow parishioners of a large urban Christian church prior to what would be a possible extensive stay in an inpatient pediatric oncology unit for high-dose induction chemotherapy. The oncologists tried to explain to the family that delaying the start of chemotherapy was risky because of the exponential growth measured on the young girl's tumor. Upon hearing that the oncologists wanted her to go directly to the hospital for treatment to be initiated that evening (most likely a high-dose, multi-drug chemotherapy treatment plan), the family left the clinic with the child in tears. The oncologist, fearful that the family may not return or may choose to delay the onset of treatment by days, repeatedly telephoned the family to return. After hearing the telephone messages that legal guardianship for mandated treatment may need to be sought to ensure adequate treatment with a known probability of response, the family admitted the teen for treatment the next day (pediatric oncology charge nurse, San Francisco Clinic, personal communication, September 2003).

CASE 5: WANTING TRADITIONAL HEALERS

A 10-year-old boy and his mother came to a busy emergency department (ED) of a large urban hospital. The child had had a moist productive cough and a fever for over two weeks. Upon questioning the child's significant past medical history, the mother reported that the child had been successfully treated for a brain tumor at the age of 2. The ED personnel discovered that the boy had a remarkably high serum white blood count (> 300,000 mL), which was a preliminary indicator of childhood leukemia. The mother became very distraught and explained to the ED staff that the child had suffered a great deal through chemotherapy and surgeries for the treatment of his brain tumor as a toddler. She said she could not bear to see him go through that again. If this was a true diagnosis, she announced to the ED staff that she would go down to rural Mexico, where her extended family was, and seek the assistance of a *curandero* (a traditional native healer or shaman found in Latin America). After being left alone behind a curtained-off ED bed while the staff contemplated what steps to take next, the mother and child left the ED AMA and went home. The ED staff became very concerned after placing several phone calls to the home requesting that she bring the boy back to the hospital for an extensive workup to rule out cancer, to no avail. The ED staff subsequently notified social services, the hospital administrator, the hospital lawyer, and finally the local county child protective agency. Two days later, the social worker accompanied a law enforcement agent to the family's home and brought the child to the hospital for imminent treatment. A court order for mandated treatment was required to ensure that the child was treated for a diagnosis of leukemia. The mother was very upset. She stayed at the bedside at all times documenting every staff member's interventions, stating that she was going to sue. Although most difficult to deal with, the mother was allowed and even encouraged to stay since she never physically obstructed the nurses administrating the treatment or became belligerent again. The child responded to the cancer treatment and was released weeks later to his mother's care. Long-term treatment was going to be required (Anonymous, personal communication, October 2003).

CASE 6: CULTURE AND TRADITION

A 2-year-old toddler was being treated for a new diagnosis of type I diabetes mellitus. The parents, faithful Muslims, requested that the child receive only insulin that was human, not pork- or beef-based. The child experienced complications during his initial hospitalization and required intravenous therapy for dehydration and ketoacidosis. The heparin used for flushing his line was a low dose anticoagulant used to keep the intravenous tubing patent. Unfortunately, the heparin was beef-based. Family members were very disappointed with the medical, nursing, and pharmacy teams as they were not notified of the option of non-animal-based pharmaceutical products beyond the human insulin. The family was very vocal about its dismay and subsequently sought and received treatment at another hospital via a different pediatric internal medicine team (ethnographic interview participant, personal communication, January 2001).

CASE 7: NOT DISCLOSING DEATHS

As reported by Belz (2019), the Body (aka "The Body of Christ") is a small fundamentalist Christian faith group founded in Attleboro, Massachusetts. The group consists of many extended families living together in a commune lifestyle. The group split from a larger bible study group in the 1970s, the Worldwide Church of God, but took with them the doctrine of suspicion of doctors and educators. Furthermore, their faith-healing doctrine rejects allopathic medical care, even disallowing the use of eyeglasses. An infant was reported to have died within the closed community due to the withholding of food over a 51-day period to comply with a prophecy received by his aunt. The group participated in social isolation, cut off outsiders, practiced home births, and avoided medical care. The father of the infant who died received a life sentence without parole (Belz, 2019).

CASE 8: SHUNNING MEDICAL CARE

In Florida, within a small evangelical Christian group, between 1996 and 1998, two children died as a direct result of the shunning of allopathic medical care. A 3-month-old died by choking to death without the family calling for medical assistance (the parents were acquitted), and a 2-year-old was stung by 432 yellow jackets. The parents of the 2-year-old allegedly waited for seven hours before calling the paramedics. Upon arrival, the child had no pulse and was not breathing. The parents were eventually charged with aggravated child abuse (Ontario Consultants on Religious Tolerance, n.d.).

CASE 9: APPLYING FAITH HEALING

Members of the Endtime Ministries have been reported to have lost several church members in several states as a result of their exclusive belief in faith healing. Five newborns died during home births (unattended by licensed practitioners), and two women died in 1990. The parents of a boy were charged with child abuse when they refused an operation for a heart tumor. The boy had lost approximately 30% of his weight, had both kidney and liver failure, and suffered the consequences of long-term malnutrition. The same family lost a newborn child from massive hemorrhaging as the parents did not seek medical treatment (Ontario Consultants on Religious Tolerance, n.d.).

CASE 10: REFUSAL BASED ON FAITH

Members of the Faith Assembly Church denied medical treatment to a 4-year-old child with an eye tumor the size of her head. The trails of blood were just the height of the young girl's head. The police discovered that the girl, who was nearly blind, used the wall to support her head and tumor as she walked room to room, leaving a streak of blood as she navigated between rooms. A neighbor reported the situation to the appropriate authorities, who then sought treatment interventions. Legal outcome of the situation was not disclosed in the report (Rick A. Ross Institute of New Jersey, n.d.).

CASE 11: USE OF ALTERNATIVE TREATMENTS

Parents of a comatose 10-year-old girl refused traditional rehabilitative treatment for their child, who suffered irreversible brain damage following prolonged seizures after a near-drowning accident. The family, after many discussions through family conferences, was told further treatments would be required if any improvements of her condition were to be attained. The family adamantly expressed a desire to administer Chinese herbs and concentrated teas via her nasogastric tube. On several occasions, the nursing staff found the father administering solutions via the tube. After continuing investigations and negotiations, the medical team supported the parents' desire to co-treat the child with traditional Chinese medicine. The parents consented to further diagnostics and interventions once they felt their concerns were heard and respected and their cultural practices were accepted as a valuable source of healing for their child (Anonymous, personal communication, October 2003).

CASE 12: VACCINE REFUSAL AND RELIGION

According to Pierik (2017), a number of religious groups refuse vaccines based on religious beliefs. In his article on religious and secular exemptions surrounding vaccine acceptance, he describes, on an international level, that Dutch Protestant-Christian congregations and their members refuse vaccines due to a perception that God predestines the fate of all people, including both prevalence of diseases and individual health states. Vaccines, according to Dutch Protestant-Christians, are "an inappropriate meddling in the work of God" (Pierik, 2017, para. 22).

CASE 13: VACCINE REFUSAL AND CULTURAL PERSPECTIVES

A strong cultural value is that of individualism. In the US, citizens often highly value the need to protect rights for themselves and their children. Being told that vaccines are mandatory can go against cultural beliefs in individuality and self-protection of rights. Some express their cultural perspectives on vaccines by making references to suspicion and apprehension, which, according to the College of Physicians of Philadelphia (2020), is fairly common among what are considered "disenfranchised communities" both the in the US and internationally. Adding to this suspicion and distrust are historical events such as the Tuskegee Syphilis Study, where southern Blacks were denied treatment for syphilis in order for the public health departments to study disease progression. Several researchers have found that the mistrust that occurred with this study has influenced African Americans' mistrust and distrust of vaccination programs. Internationally, other cultures continue to distrust vaccines based on "Western plot" theories. Culture will continue to influence vaccine acceptance and adherence.

CASE 14: VACCINE REFUSAL AND PHILOSOPHY

A six-week-old infant was being treated in the pediatric intensive care unit for a severe case of pertussis (also known as whooping cough), a bacterial infection mostly found in unvaccinated infants and young children. The parents have a 3-year-old child who attends day care with other young children. Neither the infant nor the sibling had received childhood vaccines, as the parents were self-described "conscientious objectors" to any childhood vaccines. Both parents, educated and professionally employed, diligently staying at the intensive care crib at all times, described how their community does not believe in childhood vaccines, as the risks far outweigh the benefits—risks, they state, they are not willing to take. The small infant, just extubated and now breathing on her own, will require a long course of antibiotics to fight the bacterial infection. Her parents, planning on adhering to their anti-vaccination thought process, have been invited to a full pediatric ICU multidisciplinary team meeting.

CASE 15: TREATMENT COMPROMISE SCENARIO

Raul was a 50-year-old male who was seen in a federally qualified community health center. Raul had a 10-year history of type 2 diabetes. He was Spanish-speaking, low-income, and had no health insurance. He considered himself Latinx. He worked as a gardener and had a positive family history of type 2 diabetes. Raul's HbA1c had been about 9% for the past two years despite several oral medications that he seemed to take regularly judging by his refill history. So, his provider (who did not speak Spanish) recommended insulin, which Raul refused. The provider ended the visit and charted that "the patient is noncompliant." At the next visit, Raul was seen by a bilingual, bicultural family nurse practitioner (FNP) who, after discussing his oral meds and blood sugars and lab results, said, "So I see you don't really want to take insulin. Can you tell me more about that?" Raul responded that he was very afraid of taking insulin. "Can you tell me why?" replied the FNP. Raul stated, "I know one person who took insulin and died a month later, and another friend of mine had his leg amputated." The FNP acknowledged his fears and explained that the people he was referring to could have started insulin too late, and the damage might have already been severe. However, Raul was still very reluctant, so the FNP worked out the following treatment plan with Raul: 1) They would increase the oral medications to the maximum;

and 2) If that didn't help enough, they would discuss insulin again at the next visit. The FNP explained that there is a type of insulin that is long-acting and only needs to be taken once a day (at nighttime). The same FNP saw Raul consistently every month, and on the third month he agreed to try the insulin. He started his nightly dose, and the FNP saw him again in two weeks, when she found that there was a slight improvement. She continued to see Raul at two-week intervals, and she increased the insulin dose slightly at each visit until Raul's HbA1c was down to 7%. The factors that contributed to a good outcome in this case included:

- Culturally appropriate FNP who was bilingual in English and Spanish.
- Good rapport and trust established between patient and FNP.
- FNP took the time to find out *why* the patient was afraid of insulin instead of simply labeling him "noncompliant" and writing him off as a lost cause.
- The treatment plan was a *collaboration* between the FNP and the patient.
- Frequent, intensive follow-up appointments until the patient was stable.
- Slow titration of medication to avoid and/or minimize side effects, which might having discouraged and/or made him quit.

CASE 16: ADULT REFUSAL SCENARIO

Elmer, an 81-year-old, had a long history of a bipolar disorder. He had spent most of his adult years refusing to see a physician, as his preference was to read about a potential condition and live a healthy life to prevent complications. He had never been on any medications for any health conditions and only took one acetaminophen tablet if needed. He considered himself healthy, although he had mood swings ranging from a depression that caused him to lie in bed for most of the time outside of his professional career to manic energy that caused him to spend money, sleep very few hours each night, and experience great strain on his personal and family relationships. When he turned 81, he became very fatigued and thin and was diagnosed with pheochromocytosis with high serum iron levels, requiring regular phlebotomy appointments not to damage his liver. He refused all treatment. When he was in counsel with his physician, based on his described lifestyle and moods, he was also diagnosed with bipolar disorder. He further refused to take any medications to treat his mood disorder. Describing his philosophy of distrusting both medicine and "big pharma," he noted that he did not intend to pursue preventative phlebotomies to prevent liver damage. He died at 83 from a heart attack and stroke. He had not had his blood pressure taken for over two years.

CASE 17: DEFERRED HEALTH MAINTENANCE

Deborah was a 57-year-old woman who had been deferring her colorectal cancer screening for the past seven years. She was aware that she was supposed to have had a sigmoidoscopy at age 50, but she kept putting it off because she did not really see the need for it. She had no family history of colorectal cancer that she knew of (though her biological father had left before Deborah's first birthday and not been seen since, so Deborah knew nothing about his side of the family). Deborah did not have any symptoms of colorectal cancer, and she did not really think she had any of the risk factors for it (though she couldn't have told you exactly what the risk factors were with any degree of certainty). Deborah did go to her well woman examinations, and she was up to date on her mammograms and pap smears. However, the nurse practitioner who performed her pelvic exams frequently skipped doing a rectal exam. "You don't want a rectal exam, do you?" she had said at the last visit. "I don't think I can really tell that much when I do a rectal exam, anyway," she added.

AGAINST MEDICAL ADVICE

Deborah had been struggling with obesity her whole life. She had tried every diet with little success, and she had finally gotten to the point where she was so tired of being obese that she had made the difficult decision to opt for bariatric surgery. However, there were hurdles to overcome. The large HMO that supplied her health insurance required counseling, support group visits, a psychiatric evaluation, and the loss of 10% of one's body weight prior to bariatric surgery to demonstrate commitment. In addition to all of that, the surgeon had a requirement of his own. He flatly refused to operate on anyone whose routine health maintenance was not up to date. Deborah said to him, "I'm up to date on everything. I've had my mammogram, my pap, all my immunizations are up to date. I'm good to go!" The surgeon replied, "You haven't had a colonoscopy." Deborah protested that she didn't really need one and she would be happy to sign a release declining the procedure and holding him harmless. The surgeon was unmoved. "No colonoscopy, no surgery," he said. Deborah was terribly upset. She felt no one should have the right to force her to have a procedure she didn't want. On the other hand, she did want the bariatric surgery very badly, and she had fulfilled all the other requirements. Accordingly, she reluctantly asked her primary care provider to refer her for a colonoscopy. The colonoscopy was performed, and a 3.5 cm adenocarcinoma was discovered. Deborah had to have chemo, radiation, and a bowel resection for stage III rectal cancer.

1 WHEN MEDICAL TREATMENT AND PATIENT NEEDS CLASH

Factors to Consider Regarding the Case of Deferred Health Maintenance

- The surgeon who refused to operate until all routine health maintenance was up to date literally saved Deborah's life!

- Deborah was not well educated about the importance of colorectal screening. She was unaware that colorectal cancer is the third leading cause of cancer death in women and the second leading cause of cancer death in men.

- Deborah was unaware that she *did* have many of the risk factors such as obesity, a diet high in red meat, a history of cigarette smoking, alcohol consumption, sedentary lifestyle, etc. Deborah knew nothing about her paternal family health history, so it is possible that there was a positive genetic risk, as well.

- Deborah's rectal mass would most likely have been palpable, had the clinician who performed her annual exam done a rectal examination.

- Deborah is adamant that it would be wrong to blame others for her own treatment refusal. However, when pressed, she speculates that she *might* have complied if any of her healthcare providers had pushed her to get a colonoscopy sooner.

- At the very least, Deborah's healthcare providers missed a number of opportunities (over seven years' time) to provide Deborah with some much-needed health education related to the necessity for colorectal cancer screening.

CASE 18: AN OLDER ADULT TAKING HORMONE REPLACEMENT THERAPY FOR REASONS NOT INDICATED

Cheryl is an 82-year-old widow who lives in a retirement home. She is quite active and looks younger than her age. She takes a great deal of pride in her appearance and spends a lot of time doing her hair and makeup every day. She is scornful of the older adult residents in her retirement community who must use walkers and who are unable to drive any longer. They congregate together every day after lunch and can be heard laughing, socializing, and playing games together, but Cheryl flatly refuses to join them (even though she admits to being lonely since the death of her husband three years ago). Cheryl has been taking a high dose of hormone replacement therapy (HRT) for many years, even though it may raise her odds of heart disease, breast cancer, and stroke. Her daughter-in-law (who is a breast cancer survivor) has been pressuring Cheryl to quit the HRT or at least talk to the prescribing provider about cutting down on the dose. Cheryl refuses to consider this because she believes the HRT keeps her face from being wrinkled and helps her to look younger. While this case is not an example of a treatment refusal, it does highlight the importance of elucidating how well patients understand their own medical treatment and ascertaining their associated beliefs.

CASE 19: PATIENT REFUSING IMMUNIZATIONS FOR HIMSELF AND HIS DAUGHTER

Kevin is a young man with an engaging smile. He is 23 years old and is a construction worker in a small town in Idaho. Kevin and his friends believe in a great many conspiracy theories, and he steadfastly refuses immunizations for himself and for his 18-month-old daughter. "I hate going into the clinic," Kevin says. "The nurse and the doctor are both totally judgmental. They are always trying to violate my civil liberties for refusing immunizations. It's my body, it should be

1 WHEN MEDICAL TREATMENT AND PATIENT NEEDS CLASH

my choice. They must be getting a kickback from big pharma!" he states angrily. Kevin believes that pharmaceutical companies stand to make so much money off vaccines that they regularly bribe researchers to fake their data, cover up evidence of the harmful side effects of vaccines, and inflate statistics on vaccine efficacy. Kevin believes that vaccines have dangerous side effects and that exposure to the disease itself would often be preferable to the vaccination. Further, from reading anti-vaccination blogs on the internet and talking to his friends, Kevin asserts that there is a significant amount of evidence that vaccines can hurt more than they help. "For example, by the year 2020, tens of thousands of reactions to vaccines, including deaths, have been reported. You also need to consider that these figures should be magnified tenfold, because 90% of doctors don't report adverse incidents," he adds.

In speaking with Kevin over several lengthy interviews, four overarching themes emerged: 1) Trust is a huge issue for him. He is suspicious about the scientific community, and he has great concerns about personal liberty. 2) He wants alternatives. He is hyper-focused on the chemicals in vaccines, and he would prefer the use of homeopathic remedies over vaccination. 3) Safety is a big issue for him. He has tremendous concern about immunization risk, and he perceives vaccination as being almost immoral. 4) Conspiracy is the biggest issue of all. Kevin is certain that government deliberately "hides" the information that he and his friends who do not believe in vaccination are certain to be facts.

CASE REMARKS

These are but a few of the hundreds of cases found in both in-depth interviews and past and current literature. Not all of these cases can be substantiated or confirmed, as not all websites can be deemed accurate in the reporting of the case. Some of the cases discovered in investigating sources for this book will never be brought to the public's eye, as they were resolved quietly between the family and healthcare team or between the primary physician and law enforcement, or they were not discovered by media reporters.

There is no national registry or reporting mandate for treatment refusal cases or for leaving a healthcare organization AMA. Cases including children and older adults may or may not be reported as child abuse or elder abuse, and the parents or families may or may not be indicted for child abuse, adult abuse, or neglect. The process of discovery and the follow-through, as well as the subsequent final outcome of these cases, can be quite varied.

CHAPTER 2

OVERVIEW AND REASONS FOR TREATMENT REFUSALS

Healthcare professionals administer care to children and adults suffering from injuries, disease, and disorders. When a parent refuses recommended treatment or sets treatment or diagnostic exam limitations, the situation can become strained and problematic. When adults refuse medical diagnostics or treatments, the situation becomes distressing, and the team worries as the adult leaves their care with unknown outcomes. Few healthcare professionals know exactly what to do in these situations. How does one try to educate another person and talk to the person about allopathic medical care when they want to refuse? The well-being of a child—even the survival of a child—is the ultimate concern of both parents and healthcare providers. Yet, who has the right to say what should and should not be done for either faithful and loving parents or an adult with a set mind?

In many countries, there is great cultural value placed on the autonomy of parental decisions for their children. These decisions include child-rearing, education, discipline, socialization, safety, and recreation. When it comes to medical decisions, it is generally understood that parents will supply competent healthcare for their child. For adults who refuse or will not consent to treatment, their autonomy is not questioned. Their state of mind and mental competence may be questioned, but ultimately, their autonomy is respected.

According to Clutter (2005), most people believe life has a spiritual aspect, and God does indeed exist. The influence of these beliefs on family functioning is important. In general, there have been three powerful influencing factors to medical treatment refusal: religion and religious beliefs, culture and cultural norms/practices, and what we will talk about throughout this book: one's individual or shared philosophy.

FACTORS ASSOCIATED WITH TREATMENT REFUSALS

The following sections discuss three areas associated with treatment refusal.

RELIGION

Religion and one's faith can be highly influential in life's decision-making. According to the 2018 Gallup Poll (Brenan, 2018), 72% of Americans say religion is "important" to them, and 51% report that religion is "very important." Medical care and treatment, whether diagnostic, treatment-oriented, or preventative in nature, may or may not be influenced by one's faith or religious affiliation. There are, however, over 31 religious groups who have faith doctrines that influence whether a child can receive allopathic medical treatment or whether a child or adult should have a religious service (i.e., laying on of hands, group prayer sessions or consultation or approval from a religious leader) prior to accepting allopathic medical care (Linnard-Palmer, 2006). This refusal, delay, or limitation can influence the clinical outcomes of the person's or child's health, including leading to expedited death.

The influence of spiritual beliefs on family functioning is important to keep in mind as healthcare is delivered. As adults, parents, and children experience illness, trauma, disease, separation, and changes in life, professionals should keep in mind how important those beliefs may be (Clutter, 2005). Healthcare professionals must be comfortable in assessing beliefs, religious preferences, and spiritual backgrounds and be able to use this information to help all members of the family research mutually acceptable and safe patient outcomes.

CULTURE

One's cultural background can be highly influential in health-related decision-making. Sometimes a cultural value concerning health has its own prescribed treatments. This includes traditional Chinese medicine, traditional Native American healing practices, and traditional Mexican treatments for particular disorders or states like childhood fevers. Other times, the cultural norm is to seek guidance from experienced leaders or heads of cultural or ethnic groups. It is not uncommon for Native Americans to seek counsel from tribal leaders on decisions concerning cancer treatment, symptom management, or acceptance of vaccines. According to the College of Physicians of Philadelphia (2018), culturally divergent views of treatments such as vaccines include suspicions, American ploys and plots, misunderstandings (e.g., HIV was transferred from monkeys to man via a polio vaccine), and apprehension (polio vaccines administered in Afghanistan were a ploy to sterilize Muslim populations, and in Nigeria, claims were made that vaccines were purposely contaminated to cause AIDS and sterilization and contained cancer-causing agents; Warraich, 2009), especially for disenfranchised communities.

PHILOSOPHY

Philosophy can be defined in two ways: It is the study of the fundamental nature of reality, existence, and knowledge; and it is considered a theory or attitude held by a person or organization that acts as *guiding principles* (Brown University, 2021). There is no one universal definition of the phrase "philosophical perspectives of medical treatment." There are, nevertheless, a plethora of examples of how one's philosophy has influenced the acceptance or rejection of allopathic medical care, treatments, and vaccines. Perspectives include:

- Mandating treatments or vaccines is a violation of one's individual rights to care for one's own body (Anonymous, personal communication, 2020).

- Individuals who have access to vaccines, and for whom vaccines are not contraindicated, have "a moral obligation to contribute to the realization of herd immunity . . . in spite of the fact that each individual vaccination does not significantly affect vaccinations coverage rates . . . (nor) significantly contribute to herd immunity" (Giubilini et al., 2018, p. 1).

- Parents' rights over their children's healthcare, considered parental autonomy, is not a "right" as is adults making decisions about their medical treatment. Adults' decisions may conflict with what is best for them as individuals, but parents' views "may be idiosyncratic, based on religious or other supernatural beliefs, or unreasonable" (Wilkinson & Savulescu, 2018, pp. 1–2).

According to Pierik (2017, para. 32):

In the last three decades, a vocal anti-vaccination movement has emerged, which conveys its message primarily through anti-vaccination websites. This is a multifaceted movement, including 'spiritual' or 'holistic' approaches, anthroposophist, homeopaths, and adherents of 'natural healing' and 'alternative healing.' They dispute the medical consensus that vaccines are safe and effective; moreover, they question the self-evidence with which governments provide and promote large-scale vaccination programs.

These perspectives and more will be addressed later in the book. What is most important is to learn, practice, and apply the skills of assessment and evaluation when talking to individuals or groups about philosophical perspectives that influence important medical decision-making.

It is very important not to belittle the impact of treatment decisions, either adult or pediatric, for all involved. It is most distressing for the family if treatment wishes are not honored. It is also very distressing and difficult for the healthcare professional involved to invest time-consuming and often morally distressing energy toward negotiations that frequently result in continued refusals. People want to avoid disagreements or battles over treatment decisions. It is not easy and sometimes unavoidable, yet negotiations must be attempted, especially when children are involved, so that courts, judges, and guardianships are not used as threats to secure a child's safety.

ADDITIONAL REASONS FOR TREATMENT REFUSAL

There are many reasons why parents refuse or limit treatment, whether or not they lose guardianship. Religious reasons, cultural influences, and philosophical beliefs, although the basis for this book, represent just three of the many identified reasons why parents, families, and adults say no to allopathic Western medical care.

Frequency of treatment refusal in general is well documented across childhood in literature, media, and court proceedings (Appelbaum & Roth, 1983). The exact frequency of the phenomenon of medical treatment refusal *and* subsequent loss of temporary guardianship for minors is unknown. Upon interviewing a number of nurses and physicians who have worked extensively in the field of pediatrics in large urban medical centers in California, stories of treatment refusal based on religious frameworks, cultural reasons, and other reasons abound. Examples of loss of guardianship following treatment refusal are found less frequently, demonstrating that refusal situations are often handled without the need to obtain state court intervention.

Swan (1997) reports on the deaths of children that were documented after medical care was withheld on the grounds of religious beliefs. There were 170 deaths between 1975 and 1995 in approximately 18 religious sects that object to medical intervention. As cited in Asser and Swan's 1998 research article, of the 172 children identified by referral or record searches who died from the practice and application of faith healing in lieu of medical care between 1975 and 1995, 140 fatalities were from conditions in which medical care could have provided a 90% survival rate, 18 could have had a survival rate of approximately 50%, and all but three of the rest would have probably had some clinical benefit of the application of allopathic medical care.

There are numerous powerful reasons behind parental decisions to refuse or limit medical treatment. The following list was condensed from health science and related literature of the past 21 years:

1. Religious frameworks concerning preference for prayer over medical treatments, or prior to any allopathic medical care, are found nationally and internationally.

2. Religious frameworks concerning limits on interventions such as various blood and blood product transfusion therapies, specialized diet therapies, or diagnostics have been found across America.

2 OVERVIEW AND REASONS FOR TREATMENT REFUSALS

3. Ambiguous consenting procedures by healthcare professionals seeking parental approval and signature for medical treatments, diagnostics, or procedures can lead to refusal to sign consent forms. Healthcare providers often try to rush the process of consenting for diagnostics, treatments, transfusions, or surgeries, leading parents to refuse or delay consent. This rush is often related to the hectic interdisciplinary schedule of pediatric hospital departments.

4. Conflicting or ambiguous sources of information on treatment decisions can occur. Because of the vast array of technology, it is not uncommon for parents to seek second or third opinions, which can then delay consent and/or treatments.

5. Influences on the access to sophisticated medical technology have led to fears, states of confusion, and delays in treatment consent.

6. Pressures during the treatment decision-making time frame can occur. Some religious or cultural practices warrant council by church elders, high-level church representatives, or tribal leaders, which in turn causes treatment delays.

7. Conscientious objectors to medical care or treatment exist. Some people simply do not trust or wish to apply modern, standardized medical care. Many in this category are not affiliated with any particular cultural or religious group. Some may believe that procedures are overlapping, or repeated measures are just not warranted. Sometimes they are right and sometimes they are not. This mistrust may add to the confusion.

8. Use of alternative medicine modalities rather than Western medical practices have become commonplace in the US. With the rising number of Americans who use complementary, alternative, or integrative treatments, parental desires to apply various non-Western healing methods are escalating.

9. Parental relationships with other siblings can become strained or compromised, and the sacrifice of family life (quality of life) during the demands of care for the ill child requiring treatment may be perceived to be too great. In other words, families may say "No" to a complex and expensive treatment for one child so that the quality of life of the family as a whole is not changed or is minimally impacted.

10. Cost in dollars, loss of employment for care, or inability to maintain employment during care for the ill child can all lead parents to refuse treatment.

11. Mental capabilities of parents during treatment decisions may influence consenting procedures or treatment decision-making. Illiteracy, lower educational levels, and poor comprehension abilities can influence whether a parent readily consents for medical treatments.

12. Pressures and emotional turmoil during treatment decisions may be too great.

13. Mental capabilities of children concerning treatment decisions may influence parents' treatment decisions.

14. Issues concerning best interest for the child may influence consenting procedures.

15. Concerns of quality of life for the child after complex medical treatments with little known positive outcomes may influence parental decisions.

(Information summarized from Linnard-Palmer, 2006; Linnard-Palmer & Kools, 2005; Overbay, 1996; Paris & Bell, 1993; Rhodes, 1999; Ruccione et al., 1991.)

There are probably many more reasons for treatment refusal that can be identified, as family constellation, structure, function, and decision-making power differs for each unique family system. The current scientific literature clearly describes how the healthcare system is arranged for parents to bring in their ill child; consent to prescribed

2 OVERVIEW AND REASONS FOR TREATMENT REFUSALS

diagnostic exams, pharmaceuticals, treatments, and surgeries; and allow the healthcare system to make the treatment decisions. Healthcare providers have efficient routines on which they rely on a daily basis. Most do not want these routines disrupted. Western medical systems are fast-paced; often are not concerned with religious, cultural, or philosophical individual or family needs; and tend to practice with cookie-cutter precision. When parents refuse to cooperate with the "standard" expected of hospitalized patients and their families, for whatever reason, healthcare team members can become derailed. Pressure on the parents to cooperate can lead to the creation of future dissonance and departure.

The emotional impact of having an ill child is monumental. Parents are often not in the right state of mind or prepared emotionally to consent to imminent medical interventions for their child. There is no one solution for this situation, as early interventions for most childhood illnesses produce better outcomes. Yet, when treatments are applied without full parental involvement and consent, tragic consequences can emerge from applying interventions against the family's beliefs, convictions, or principles. Critical concern, based on data for each situation, is needed.

CHAPTER 3

CHILDHOOD VACCINES, HESITANCY, AND REFUSALS

Since the inception of childhood vaccines (also called *immunizations*), parents have expressed concerns about the safety of the contents and short- and long-term consequences. Most parents will not question the merit of childhood vaccines whose purpose is to prevent select childhood illnesses that can cause significant morbidity, injury, and sometimes death. Questioning vaccines does not always mean parents are going to refuse. They may have particular concerns that they have heard about or read about. Healthcare providers must be the most trusted source of information for parents, and language should be used that denotes confidence, accuracy, and an assumption that parents will consent.

The term *"anti-vax" parents* is used to describe those who decide not to vaccinate their children. They tend to be Caucasian, higher-than-average income earners, have a college education, and are typically mothers (Reich, 2019). Anti-vax parents have described their reactions to vaccines as disgust, suspicion, and confusion, with dismissal based on an anti-science perspective.

According to McKee and Bohannon (2016), there are four overarching reasons that parents refuse childhood vaccines. These reasons can and do vary widely among parents. The four categories are personal beliefs, religious reasons (this includes philosophical reasons), safety concerns, and a desire for more information from healthcare providers.

TYPES OF VACCINES

There are currently five general types of vaccines administered and two new advancements still in the works (Grimes, 2020; HHS.gov, 2020; Linnard-Palmer & Coats, 2010, 2021; WHO, 2020, para. 2):

1. **Live virus vaccines** (also called *live-attenuated* or *weakened*) is where whole viral material is manipulated to manufacture vaccines with a weakened strain of the virus. This weakened strain mimics the virus and causes a strong and effective launch of antibodies against the pathogen. When this type of manufacturing occurs, only one dose of the vaccine may be required. Immunocompromised patients or those of any age who have had an organ transplant and take anti-rejection medications cannot receive this type of vaccine. Examples include oral polio, nasal flu, rotavirus, measles, mumps, rubella (MMR), and varicella vaccines. Parents can ask for alternatives. Internationally, this form is not used often due to the need for refrigeration up to the point of administration. Other examples include smallpox, yellow fever, some rotavirus, and some MMR combined vaccines.

3 CHILDHOOD VACCINES, HESITANCY, AND REFUSALS

2. **Whole vaccines** are inactivated and killed whole organisms where both the internal structures and the surface proteins are used as stimulants to promote an immune response. Formalin, thimerosal, heat, or phenols may be used to kill the microbe. Multiple vaccine doses are needed. Examples are anthrax, cholera, rabies, typhoid, and inactivated polio vaccines.

3. **Polysaccharide conjugate vaccines** are a form where sugars from the bacteria are bonded to portions of another microbe—like a bacteria protein or *capsid* (bacterial casing located around the microbe). Other terms for this technology beside polysaccharide are *subunit* and *conjugate* vaccines. These cause a strong immune response and often target building antibodies against specific parts of the microbe. Boosters may be required for continued effectiveness. Examples include HIB, Hep B, HPV, shingles, and meningococcal vaccines.

4. **Toxoid vaccines** use only a harmful product produced by the microbe, a toxin, to create immunity against only the toxin part of the germ, not the entire germ itself. Examples include diphtheria and tetanus, which require boosters.

5. **Recombinant vaccines** use recombinant technology to produce a genetically altered organism with manufactured proteins that match closely with the microbe but are incapable of causing the disease. Both *Haemophilus influenzae* and pneumococcal pneumonia may be administered using this newer technology.

6. Two new technologies remain under study: **recombinant vector vaccines** (also called *platform-based* vaccines), which are effective in teaching the immune system to fight the targeted microbe, and **DNA vaccines**, which are strong, inexpensive to produce, and provide lasting immunity. According to the World Health Organization (WHO, 2020, para. 2):

    > Recently a radical new approach to vaccination has been developed. It involves the direct introduction into appropriate tissues of a plasmid

containing the DNA sequence encoding the antigen(s) against which an immune response is sought, and relies on the in situ production of the target antigen . . . advantages over traditional approaches, including the stimulation of both B- and T-cell responses, improved vaccine stability, the absence of any infectious agents and the relative ease of large-scale manufacture . . . immune responses in animals have been obtained using genes from a variety of infectious agent, including influenza virus, hepatitis B virus, lymphocytic choriomeningitis virus, malarial parasites and mycoplasmas.

7. Most recently, the new vaccines created for the COVID-19 pandemic (SARS-C0V-2) by Moderna (mRNA-1273 vaccine) and Pfizer-BioNTech (BNT162b2 vaccine) use a technique whereby lipid nanoparticles and a **messenger RNA** deliver information to the human macrophage, or viral-specific T cells—DNA to create a protein that is expressed on the cell (90–95% efficacy). This expressed protein, called a *spike* protein, triggers a massive construction of antibodies against the COVID-19 virus, which then provides protection from the disease. Once the protein message is delivered to the host cell DNA, the message is used only once and then broken down by the cell and destroyed (Centers for Disease Control and Prevention [CDC], 2021c, para. 2).

The alternative type of approved COVID-19 vaccines manufactured by AstraZeneca, Johnson & Johnson, and Gam-COVID-vac (Sputnik V) use a different form of technology to result in antibody production. These companies use DNA delivered by a non-replicating adenovirus (recombinant) vector system causing the encoding of the SARS-CoV-2 spike protein to produce neutralizing antibodies (70–91% efficacy). According to Teijaro & Farber (2021), this type of technology is currently being used effectively in the Ebola vaccine.

3 CHILDHOOD VACCINES, HESITANCY, AND REFUSALS

Contrary to many people's concerns, the use of mRNA vaccine technology is not new to science. Used for many decades in animal studies, mRNA vaccines have been investigated for efficacy with rabies, Zika, and cytomegalovirus infections. Future hopes for this technology include the use of a single mRNA vaccine for coverage for several infections within one injection. Currently, oncology studies have been using mRNA technology to fight specific targeted cancer cells (CDC, 2021c, paras. 8–11).

SUMMARY OF PARENTAL CONCERNS TO VACCINES AND SUGGESTED RESPONSES

The following presents common vaccine concerns expressed by parents and subsequent suggested responses:

Concern: There are too many shots given at one time, and this can harm my child.

Response: There is no evidence to date that receiving more than one shot overwhelms the immune system of a healthy child.

Concern: The vaccines are produced in mass for the financial benefit of pharmaceutical companies.

Response: Vaccines are manufactured by specific pharmaceutical companies, but they are produced to reduce the incidence and prevalence of childhood diseases.

Concern: Vaccines can cause the illness.

Response: Vaccines come in several forms, including small particles of *antigen* (proteins or genetic material), or they are created by a process known as *attenuated* (killed).

Concern: Vaccines can be done at any time, so refusing now means I can change my mind later.

Response: Delaying childhood vaccines, according to a set schedule with multi-dosing to maximize antibody production, may result in the child acquiring the disease.

Concern: Vaccines are more dangerous than the disease they prevent.

Response: The diseases vaccines prevent are dangerous and can cause significant injury (deafness from measles and brain damage from pneumococcal meningitis) and even death; there is no way to tell if an infant will have a mild case or a severe case.

Concern: Vaccines are linked to autism, deafness, seizures, asthma, and auto-immune diseases.

Response:

- There is no current research that links childhood vaccines to these concerns. The onset of autistic symptoms coincides with the timing of several vaccine series in young children, but no connection has been found (Eggertson, 2010).
- A link between autism and childhood vaccines has been heavily researched. No scientific conclusions have been found to link the two. Unfortunately, in 1998, an article in the medical journal *The Lancet* was published linking the MMR vaccine to the development of autism. No less than 20 epidemiological investigations have been completed since that study was released, and no connection can be made between the vaccine,

3 CHILDHOOD VACCINES, HESITANCY, AND REFUSALS

thimerosal and MMR, and autism. Parents with vaccine concerns may still bring up the original *Lancet* article.

Concern: Preservatives such as *thimerosal* (mercury compound) are harmful.

Response:

- Thimerosal is a water-soluble, crystalline powder added to vaccines historically as a preservative (CDC, 2020c).
- Thimerosal does not stay in the body a long time, so it does not build up and reach harmful levels. When thimerosal enters the body, it breaks down to ethylmercury and thiosalicylate, which are readily eliminated (CDC, 2020c).
- Thimerosal was taken out of childhood vaccines in the United States in 2001. Thimerosal is only found in multi-dose influenza vaccines; infants and children receive single dose vaccines and are not exposed to thimerosal (CDC, 2020c).
- California law prohibits administering mercury-containing vaccines to pregnant women or to children younger than 3. All routine vaccines are available in formulations that meet the law.
- Current research has not found a link between thimerosal and autism or any other significant health concern.
- Families can ask for childhood vaccines without thimerosal.

Concern: Other materials in vaccines are unsafe.

Response:

- *Adjuvants*, or *enhancers*, are used to help develop a better immune response (aluminum salts), sugars and gelatin are used as stabilizers, egg proteins may be found as residual cell culture materials, and residual inactivating ingredients such as formaldehyde are used to kill microbes.

- Aluminum salts specifically are added in many vaccines to increase and improve the vaccine's effectiveness; this is especially true for combined vaccines into one injection.

Concern: Serious side effects like Guillain-Barre syndrome, seizure disorders, encephalitis, encephalopathy, and hypotonic/hyporesponsiveness episodes can happen.

Response:

- Guillain-Barre disorder can occur, although very rarely, when after the vaccine is administered, the child's body attacks not only the vaccine material but also the nervous system, which can cause temporary paralysis. This can last a short time or up to a few weeks, requiring the child to be transferred and cared for in an intensive care unit. Meningococcal vaccines, tetanus-containing vaccines, and some influenza vaccines have been associated with this condition. Although quite rare, parents need education on the more frequent complications, some very severe, associated with the diseases these vaccines prevent (CDC, 2020a).

- Encephalitis and encephalopathy, which is the inflammation and swelling of brain tissue, are rare complications in infants. Documentation states that lethargy alternating with screaming, elevated fevers, and progressive brain injury are rare and associated with the older style MMR, tetanus-containing, DTP, DTwP, and DTaP vaccines. Although most countries now use acellular DTaP which is safer, the DTwP vaccine is still used in the developing world. According to the Institute for Vaccine Safety (2018), people who become naturally infected with the mumps virus (wild type) can experience encephalitis, although rarely. There is no current evidence that the vaccines used now for varicella, meningococcal, or hepatitis B have "mechanistic evidence of quality" to show an association with either encephalitis or encephalopathy (Institute for Vaccine Safety, 2018).

3 CHILDHOOD VACCINES, HESITANCY, AND REFUSALS

- Hypotonic/hyporesponsive episodes are very rare but serious. After a vaccine is administered, mostly with DTP, DPwP, and DTaP vaccines, the child may suddenly become hypotonic lasting a few minutes to a few hours. CPR may be required, and the child should be hospitalized. Parents need to understand that the rarity of this condition does not overrule the serious consequences of a child having the diseases the vaccines are given to prevent (Vigo et al., 2017).

Concern: Natural immunity is better than the immunity that comes from vaccines.

Response: Not with the complexities of the diseases vaccines prevent. Natural immunity can be "natural," which is what we are born with; "active," from exposure to a pathogen; "passive," from antibodies passing across the placenta from mother to fetus; or by injected antibody preparations such as the rabies vaccine or snake anti-venom.

Concern: If I don't complete a series, my child will have partial coverage.

Response: A full set of vaccines is required for disease prevention during childhood.

Concern: I have religious objections to using aborted fetus tissue in the creation and production of vaccines.

Response: Parents may object to the MMR vaccine as, originally, aborted human fetus tissue and gelatins from animals may be used in the production of this vaccine. According to Children's Hospital of Philadelphia (2020, pp. 1–2):

> Varicella chickenpox and rubella (the "R" in the MMR vaccine), hepatitis A, and one preparation of rabies vaccine are all made by growing the viruses in fetal embryo fibroblast cells. Fibroblast cells are the cells needed to hold

skin and other connective tissue together. The fetal embryo fibroblast cells used to grow vaccine viruses were first obtained from elective termination of two pregnancies in the early 1960s. These same embryonic cells obtained from the early 1960s have continued to grow in the laboratory and are used to make vaccines today. No further sources of fetal cells are needed to make these vaccines.

Furthermore:

Almost all cells die after they have divided a certain number of times; scientifically, this number is known as the Hayflick limit. For most cell lines, including fetal cells, it is around 50 divisions; however, because fetal cells have not divided as many times as other cell types, they can be used longer. In addition, because of the ability to maintain cells at very low temperatures, such as in liquid nitrogen, scientists are able to continue using the same fetal cell lines that were isolated in the 1960s.

Concern: Breastfeeding and healthy diet/lifestyle will prevent these childhood diseases, or at least decrease the chance of acquiring them.

Response: It is true that healthy eating, healthy lifestyles, and prolonged breastfeeding can help with illness prevention, but they will not prevent the acquisition of severe childhood infections.

Concern: If others are vaccinated, I do not need to vaccinate my child.

Response: Vaccines work best at a population level. The more children who receive vaccines, the more protection there is for others. If you look at rubella, a relatively mild disease in children, pregnant mothers who are exposed can have newborns who have birth defects, are miscarried, or who are blind or deaf. The term *herd immunity* is used to denote the resistance of contagion of a disease if a high proportion of people are vaccinated and thus immune. This concept does

3 CHILDHOOD VACCINES, HESITANCY, AND REFUSALS

not ensure a single child will be immune and thus safe from contracting the disease (CDC, 2010, 2020c; Linnard-Palmer & Coats, 2010, 2021).

Concern: The safety of the COVID-19 vaccines has not been fully determined.

Response: The mRNA vaccines and the non-replicating adenovirus (recombinant) vector system vaccine (the two types of vaccines currently approved for use) were tested on over 100,000 people enrolled in trial studies to demonstrate efficacy. Data generated in these studies show evidence that allowed an expedited vaccine production and disseminated distribution (Teijaro & Farber, 2021).

VACCINE HESITANCY

Vaccine hesitancy is a relatively new term used to denote parental concerns that are not strong enough to refuse vaccines altogether but that cause a delay due to doubts and fears. Vaccine hesitancy is considered to be on a "continuum of vaccine acceptance ranging from refusing all, refuse but unsure, delay/refuse some, accept but unsure, to accept all" (Grimes, 2020, p. 8). Globally, vaccine hesitancy is also defined as refusal or reluctance to vaccinate children despite access and availability (Akoum, 2019). According to McKee and Bohannon (2016), the majority of parents who refuse to vaccinate their children due to religious beliefs outnumber those who have hesitancy from overall concerns, "and it is very difficult to dissuade these individuals from views against immunization" (para. 4). In 2019, WHO declared vaccine hesitancy as one of the 10 most concerning global health threats (Akoum, 2019). According to Grimes (2020), one of the main precepts of vaccine hesitancy is that people are repeatedly exposed to incorrect statements about vaccines. They then sway toward falsehood despite knowing better and accept the falsehood subconsciously by hearing the falsehood via repetition. This can all contribute to vaccine hesitancy or refusal.

According to the World Health Organization as stated by WHO.org (2008) found in Grimes (2019): The best way to address those who participate in the antivaccination movement is to refute wrong allegations as early as possible using scientifically valid data. In Grimes' book, the challenge of addressing the antivaccination movement has been around since the time of Jenner*. Unfortunately, antivaccinators do not always accept science.

LAWS AND EXEMPTIONS RELATED TO CHILDHOOD VACCINES

Vaccine-preventable diseases (VPDs) have been closely monitored by the federal government since the early 1800s, when smallpox vaccines were first available (College of the Physicians of Philadelphia, 2018). Federal guidelines have been influenced by research collected and disseminated by the CDC. There are currently no federal laws concerning mandates for childhood vaccinations, only strong suggestions, especially when there have been epidemics (such as the 1,282 cases of measles in 2019 as reported by CDC, 2021b). Each state has the jurisdiction to establish criteria and create laws that govern which vaccines are required for children who are entering public and private schools and what are considered exemptions from receiving childhood vaccines. Federal organizations have compiled information on state laws concerning vaccination programs and exemptions, but federal organizations do not provide laws or mandates concerning childhood vaccinations. The CDC describes this process as working closely with private partners and state public health departments to suggest, sustain, and monitor the safety of vaccines and vaccine laws (CDC, 2018). Interesting to note, research has shown that vaccine exemp-

---

*Jenner is considered by many to be the "father" of vaccinations in the Western world. In 1757 in Gloucester, he was the first to give an 8-year-old boy named James Phipps an inoculation with smallpox. After developing a mild case of smallpox, he was considered immune to the disease (historyofvaccines.org, 2021).

3 CHILDHOOD VACCINES, HESITANCY, AND REFUSALS

tions cluster geographically, leading to outbreaks in specific communities (Omer et al., 2008; Wang et al., 2014).

The greatest influencing factor for federal recommendations for state laws is outbreaks of VPDs. As of May 2019, seven states had 10 separate and accountable measles outbreaks and at least 880 confirmed cases and thus broke the validation of the 2000 declaration that measles was eradicated in the US (CDC, 2020b). In 2014 in the Amish community of Ohio, there were 383 cases of measles (Shen, 2019). Measles can kill infants, children, and adults (Johns Hopkins Medicine, 2020).

The protection against VPDs has had an interesting history (CDC, 2016b; Shen, 2019):

- In 1796, the first immunization was created against smallpox, and in 1850 it became mandatory. Smallpox possibly began in the Egyptian Empire in the third century BC and was spread by very early trade routes. The first process to prevent the spread was by scratching or inhaling material in the nose from smallpox sores or pustules (CDC, 2016b).
- In 1905 the Supreme Court upheld state law requiring adults over 21 to be vaccinated against smallpox, as the disease was considered a public health and safety issue. The Court rejected any argument that this mandate violated liberty.
- In 1967, the WHO declared the commitment to eradicate smallpox, and in 1980, the WHO declared smallpox eradicated as the global vaccine effort had wiped out the virus.
- As of 2021, 16 states continue to provide exemptions for philosophical reasons, 45 states and Washington, DC provide exemptions for religious objections, and all states provide exemptions for medical reasons (National Conference of State Legislatures, 2020; Shen, 2019).

- "While compulsory vaccination requirements have faced legal challenges since Jacobsen v. Massachusetts [1905 case concerning mandatory smallpox vaccines for adults] and Zucht v. King [1922 case concerning exclusion from school without vaccines], courts have consistently rejected these challenges and given considerable deference to the use of the states' police power to require immunizations to protect the public health" (Shen, 2019, p. 2).

- All 50 states now have exemptions for children with allergies to components found in vaccines, children with immune-compromised states, and children who have had significant adverse reactions to vaccines. Public and private schools require childhood immunizations, as do daycare programs and infant care programs. The requirements are identical for vaccine schedules and exemptions, regardless of the type of daycare or school (CDC, 2018). Many sources state that a good way to reduce the need for exemptions is to have "stronger healthcare practices such as more in-depth discussions with hesitant parents and establishing vaccination as the default . . . to improve vaccine coverage rates" (Opel & Omer, 2015, pp. 303–304). The CDC suggests the combination of three efforts: requirement of documentation for exemption requests from parents, stronger requirements for receiving exemptions, and stronger enforcement and monitoring of received requests (CDC, 2016a).

- Under the US federalist system, general authority of vaccine laws remains under state government, as Congress only has the power to legislate what is confined to the powers described in the Constitution (Shen, 2019). States provide governing for vaccines for school attendance, select healthcare workers, and during public health emergencies (Shen, 2019, p. 2):

    Pursuant to the principles of federalism, the Supreme Court has interpreted the Tenth Amendment

3 CHILDHOOD VACCINES, HESITANCY, AND REFUSALS

to prevent the federal government from commandeering or requiring state officers to carry out federal directives. In the context of vaccination, this principle prevents Congress from requiring states or localities to pass mandatory vaccination laws, but it does not impede Congress from using its Spending Clause authority to provide incentives (in the form of federal grants) to states to enact laws concerning vaccination.

CHAPTER 4

PEDIATRIC HEALTHCARE, ETHICS, AND CHILDREN'S RIGHTS

Pediatric healthcare can be divided into five distinctly different areas. Each of these care arenas can be influenced by parents' perspectives, beliefs, and cultural norms. Each experience is unique for every family, all of whom have unique needs:

1. Well-child care and health promotion education for normal growth and development
2. Ongoing early disease and illness detection during routine community screenings (vision, hearing,

scoliosis, pediculosis, dental hygiene, child abuse and neglect, failure to thrive, and emotional distress)
3. Acute care of sudden illness needs, with interventions such as surgical procedures or antibiotics for an infection
4. Chronic care, in which a child is supported throughout childhood and adolescence during exacerbations of chronic conditions (cystic fibrosis, cancer, or diabetes)
5. Palliative, hospice, or comfort care when aggressive treatments are no longer indicated, and the focus is on symptom management and support for end-of-life care

Pediatric healthcare is complex; a child may be seen by more than one traditional pediatrician and by specialty pediatricians. The child may encounter advanced practice nurses—such as clinical nurse specialists and nurse practitioners, community health or public health nurses, and school nurses—all of whom deliver care in diverse settings. A child may be followed by a social service specialist, a developmental specialist, an academic support person, or some other group of care specialists who provide family support and resources. All of these disciplines may find that their services are influenced by the family's religious beliefs or cultural norms. It is imperative that these groups are aware of how influential belief systems can be on all areas of family functioning and a child's life.

CHILDREN'S RIGHTS

The concept of child rights is a relatively new concept in American history. In the US, animals achieved legally protected rights against cruelty prior to children receiving those rights. It was not until the early 1900s that children's rights for legal protection against work injuries and laws were established that limited the hours and conditions of child labor. According to a professor of nursing at the Dominican University of California who is a healthcare historian (personal communication, 2006), a New York lawyer was the first American to pursue legislation for child rights. The story goes that in 1905, the lawyer came upon a child who was chained to a fence while both parents went to work. From the parents' perspective, chaining the socially isolated child to the fence was the only way to keep him "safe" (never mind the exposure to the elements and acts of human cruelty). Greatly moved by this case, the lawyer immediately went to work to secure children's legal rights to protection from harm.

Parents have the constitutional right to autonomously raise their children. The US Constitution specifies that parents have the right to raise their children in relation to discipline and education. The Constitution does not, however, endow parents with the right to withhold essential medical interventions or screenings on the grounds of religious or cultural beliefs. Thus, the dichotomy between healthcare professionals and parents with distinct and influential beliefs occurs because of the desire to provide care for children while respecting parental autonomy.

According to Radcliffe (2018), parents can use much discretion in deciding what medical care their children receive, but in some instances the case could be made that refusing care could constitute neglect.

The United Nations Committee on the Rights of the Child monitors states' compliance with international guidelines and laws passed by the UN. This work is overseen by the Office of the United Nations High Commissioner for Human Rights (see www.ohchr.org/EN/pages/home.aspx). These guidelines endow all children with reasonable and appropriate rights, including medical care; however, the UN database of articles does not specifically address medical treatment refusal by parents.

Flannery (1995) describes how several Supreme Court decisions have shown that parents have what is considered a constitutional right to "bring up children," yet another Supreme Court decision held that parents have a constitutional right to make medical decisions for their children "absent of finding of abuse or neglect" (p. 9).

In 1944, the Supreme Court ruled that "the right to practice religion freely does not include liberty to expose . . . a child . . . to ill health or death. Parents may be free to become martyrs themselves, but it does not follow that they are free . . . to make martyrs of their children before the children reach the age of full and legal discretion when they can make that choice for themselves" (Prince v. Massachusetts, 321 US 158, 166, 1944). As presented in Radcliffe (2018), Efthimios Parasidis, a professor of law and public health at Ohio State University, said, "The U.S. values religious freedom to the point where states are willing to grant parents the right to refuse even life-saving medical treatments for their children if the parents can show that there's a religious tenet that would be violated by administering the treatment" (para. 6).

Adults have the right to refuse medical treatments because they have been granted self-determination. Children, however, are not considered autonomous and can neither give informed consent nor refuse treatment. Courts will at times override parents' decisions to refuse treatment based on the state child abuse or neglect laws (Fox, 1990). In Radcliffe (2018), Dr. Arthur Caplan, a bioethics professor at New York University, stated, "You need to keep in mind that parents are trying to do what's best for their kids . . . they are not doing this because they hate their kids or want to harm them" (para. 11).

Historically, parents' rights over their children's lives were considered absolute. Now, in relation to withholding necessary medical treatment, parents have limits. According to Fox (1990), "A county court in New York ruled that when parents' religious beliefs interfere with a child's right to live, the child's right is paramount, and the religious doctrine must give way" (p. 136). The right to refuse medical treatment for children is obviously a very complex phenomenon that has evolved over history.

4 PEDIATRIC HEALTHCARE, ETHICS, AND HUMAN RIGHTS

There are three legal bases for the right of an adult to refuse treatment (Rhodes & Miller, 1984):

1. The common law right to freedom from nonconsensual invasion of bodily integrity, embodied in the informed consent doctrine and the law of battery
2. The constitutional right of privacy
3. The constitutional right to freedom of religion

These are widely accepted historical principles used when the person of concern is an adult. When the person of concern is a child, these laws do not apply. Under certain circumstances, when competent adults are making healthcare decisions for minors that deviate from expected medical treatment application, courts have found it necessary to view the state's interest as outweighing those of the treatment decision-maker and have ordered treatment to take place. This seems to be in direct conflict with the three legal bases for refusal as described above. Yet, when the minor is in a life-threatening situation, the courts have overridden the decision-making rights of the parent or guardian. "Because decision-makers have an obligation to act in the best interests of the minor or incompetent adult, they must provide necessary (medical) treatment" (Rhodes & Miller, 1984, p. 216). Discretion to decline treatment is limited to situations where the treatment is elective or not likely to be beneficial. The duty to provide necessary treatment to minors is reinforced in all states by legislation concerning abused or neglected minors. This duty facilitates state intervention to provide needed assistance.

The state's authority to act as a guardian for children who are unable to make healthcare decisions for themselves is deeply entrenched in the history of 20th-century laws. Via physician requests, states may seek to protect a child by removing the child from their present custodian to another and intervene on the minor's behalf to ensure that the child is given necessary medical treatments. This is the case when the custodian, a parent or legal guardian, has been deemed unreasonable in their refusal to supply medical treatment based on religious or other grounds (Humber & Almedar, 2000; Neely, 1998).

No other more precise quote could be found in the literature than the one by Ruth Macklin as she and the Committee of Bioethics of the American Academy of Pediatrics (1988, p. 169) stated:

> Parents have the right to consent to care for their dependent children; they do not have a co-equal right to refuse care for their dependent children (Family Court Act Sections 233). Parents do not have the right to deny minor children transfusions that are deemed medically necessary. In the event that a parent withholds consent for (blood) transfusion, the hospital administration must be contacted immediately and asked to seek a court order for transfusion. In the event that medical judgment holds any delay to be immediately life-threatening to the child, (the) transfusion should be given. The boundary between parental freedom in child rearing and the interest—or even basic rights—of the child is unclear. The limits to parental decision making for children are uncertain, but it is widely accepted that parents generally will make decisions that do not directly threaten the welfare of their children. Tradition, social forces, and the belief systems shape the limits of acceptable nurturance, or parental imperatives and privileges, and even of physical force used in the discipline of children. These of course change with time. However, the constitutional guarantees of freedom of religion do not sanction harming another person in the practice of one's religion, and they do not allow religion to be a legal defense when one harms another.

4 PEDIATRIC HEALTHCARE, ETHICS, AND HUMAN RIGHTS

ETHICS

The application of ethical principles must be considered when discussing parental treatment decisions leading to either the refusal or limitation of children's basic healthcare needs. Four main ethical principles have been identified at stake within the dilemma of withholding or limiting medical treatment to children. These principles include (Fox, 1990; Gillon, 1994; IOM, 2003):

1. **Autonomy:** the insistence that all persons have intrinsic worth and therefore self-determination including both the right to decide medical treatment and religious freedoms and regarding choices about one's life and body

2. **Beneficence:** basic healthcare assumptions that include both promoting welfare as well as "acts of mercy and kindness" and the obligation to provide care that improves health

3. **Non-maleficence:** considered a greater obligation than beneficence referring to not inflicting evil or harm, and avoiding harm

4. **Justice:** the concern of fairness or impartiality and the avoidance of discrimination.

Longstanding ethical doctrines pertaining to parental rights in the care of their children include parental autonomy, parens patriae, best interest, and substituted judgment (Cushings, 1982). See the nearby sidebar for a discussion of each of these important doctrines.

Parental Rights Ethical Doctrines

Parental autonomy is a constitutionally protected right, or personal liberty right, within the 19th Amendment that pertains to procreation, marriage, child-rearing, and education. Pediatric healthcare professionals, in general, highly respect parental autonomy and will not interfere with how a parent chooses to raise their child as long as abuse, neglect, or human suffering is not identified. It is within their scope of practice for pediatric healthcare professionals to offer parenting guidelines and support so that a family is cohesive and well-adjusted to the social circumstances and culture in which that family lives. It is, nevertheless, an important professional duty to assess for effective parenting skills and identify early family crises or situations where a child is placed at risk. It then becomes the legal duty of a pediatric healthcare professional to intervene and possibly report the consequences of the risk (such as abuse or neglect) to the appropriate authorities.

Parens patriae, **Latin for "parent of the country,"** is a state's right and duty to protect children and to act as the decision-maker when needed. This right means healthcare providers are required to report all cases of child abuse or neglect. Once reported to state authorities, decisions are in the hands of those authorities (i.e., child protective agencies).

Best interest doctrine is a requirement of a court to consider subjective and objective evidence when evaluating a minor's best welfare. Several data sources can be used.

Substituted judgment is a court's determination, on behalf of an incompetent individual, of what choice the individual would make if the individual was competent. This is considered more subjective than the best interest doctrine.

The application of these ethical principles and doctrines might be needed when parents refuse medical treatment. One concern is the interference of the courts to become a decision-making body, therefore leaving a family, specifically a parent, unable to decide what is right for their child. This leaves the parent unable to direct the child's life, including applying cultural norms and practices, or religious doctrines or beliefs.

The second concern in applying ethical principles and doctrines encompasses determination of what is really best for the child, which could mean taking away the right of the parents to adhere to their religious doctrines. This conflict is seen in the historical writing of Fox (1990, p. 138):

> The result of the violation of a deeply held, long standing religious conviction can be devastating. Pope John Paul II reportedly described forcing someone to violate his or her conscience as the most painful blow inflicted on human dignity.

There can be no doubt how powerful this ethical dilemma is for both the family members, who want to adhere to their religious faith or cultural norms, and members of the healthcare team, who must live with the consequences of their actions—not just specifically their conscience, but also the consequences on the child and family. Both legal and ethical doctrines shed light on these dilemmas and allow all people involved to begin to understand what the dilemma encompasses and move toward an ethical conclusion or an ethical answer.

According to Catlin (1997), the phenomenon of treatment refusal or limitation of treatment in the pediatric population places the members of the healthcare team into a "classical ethical dilemma" (p. 289). Two competing harms have been described by Catlin as: 1) the articulated harm of a child in a critical condition that may be worsened by withholding medical treatment; and 2) the more explicated harm that takes place when a parent's decision-making is overruled or legally supervened. Healthcare team members, including nurses, have been taught to respect personal differences. Diverse races, cultures, ethnicities, and religious frameworks are aspects of client care that nurses consider. The participation in this ethical dilemma between divergent frameworks in healthcare situations can lead to personal distress for the nurse. Nurses, for instance, have been taught to always be supportive advocates for patients and families, yet the petition for legally mandated temporary guardianship to enforce medical treatments may be perceived as in direct conflict with the notion of parent and family advocacy.

Much has been written about the advocacy role inherent in the practice of nursing. Yet, some of the most crucial advocacy situations carry a risk factor, particularly in relation to the care of children. Can one be a professional advocate when the basic support for religious preferences and application is prohibited? Many questions remain unanswered, and neither the medical nor nursing science literature demonstrates great inquiry into this debate. According to Catlin (1997, p. 289):

> Nurses recognize that one of the greatest joys that exist in parenting is sharing with one's children the values of family traditions and culture. Christians baptize their children, Jews circumcise their males, Muslims fast at Ramadan, and Hindus have ceremonies of anointing with oils and spices, and rarely do nurses interfere with closely held, faith-based customs.

Being an advocate for activities and practices that cause no harm or human suffering is easy. Being an advocate for the application of religious or cultural practices that lead to withholding essential healthcare is difficult, or maybe contrary to safe practice. Glover and Rushton (1995, p. 5) succinctly describe this difficult ethical debate:

> We may claim certainty about medical facts, or about what our faith traditions require as a way of avoiding difficult

discussion and decisions. If we resort to unilateral decision making—by professionals or parents—we risk cutting moral dialogue short and seriously misconstruing our shared obligations to our children.

Because philosophical analysis rather than empirical inquiry has guided much of the current activity in bioethics, research in clinical practice is greatly needed. The methods of ethnographic research support the inquiry of the impact of treatment refusal on the parent, child, family, clergy, and healthcare professional. In the second half of this book, space is dedicated to the presentation of ethnographic research methods that explore the impact of parental medical treatment refusal, with or without loss of guardianship, on the experiences of all involved.

CHAPTER 5

LEGAL IMPLICATIONS AND CONSENT: INFORMED CONSENT, ASSENT, AND PARENTAL PERMISSION

A question contemplated by members of pediatric health science disciplines is whether children have the capacity to participate in collaborative decision-making concerning healthcare and treatment decisions. Research has shown that when children's developmental stage, not solely their chronological age, is considered, then their input can be a sincere influence on treatment decisions. This is a critical thought when parents are refusing or limiting medical treatment based on *their* religious beliefs, which may or may not be shared by the child. Pediatricians and pediatric nurses should assess the child's ability to give input and value the child's verbalized wishes as a component to the treatment trajectory.

INFORMED CONSENT

To illustrate a child's ability to give input into treatment decisions, note the following example. A nurse recounts a case of a 9-year-old boy—nearing his 10th birthday—who is refusing treatment for a recurring brain tumor. Tommy had been diagnosed with a rapid growing supratentorial brain tumor at the age of 7. At that time, the family requested treatment to be delayed in order to have a team of church members assemble to pray for their son's healing. Reluctant to support this delay, the pediatrician and pediatric neurosurgeon were able to convince both parents to consent to treatment and had persuaded the influential grandparents to offer their support during the initial treatments. The parents, now willing, consented for further treatment. Tommy, however, vehemently refused to undergo surgery and chemotherapy again. The child's quality of life was affected by his initial treatments three years prior. The child articulately expressed his wishes not to experience chemotherapy and surgical interventions again. Ultimately, he did receive treatments for this second episode of tumor regrowth, but the discerning medical team gave the child time to express his fears, concerns, and wishes. As it turned out, his concerns were not associated with the actual treatments but rather focused on whether he would receive adequate symptom management and relief from nausea, pain, and sleep disturbances leading to chronic fatigue.

The American Academy of Pediatrics (AAP) published an initial policy statement in 1976 discussing the legal concept of "informed consent" in pediatric medical practice. Historically, authority to make medical decisions once lay solely in the hands of physicians. Now, in response to continuing complex social changes, physicians must ask permission and consent from their patients, as patients have the right to decide. Patients have the right to know all options for treatments, all available diagnostic options, and the risks and benefits associated with each. Parents also have a right to this knowledge when children require medical treatment, but they do not have the right to withhold life-sustaining or lifesaving treatments based on their cultural or religious groups, nor do they have the right to cause harm (AAP.org, Committee on Bioethics, 2016).

ASSENT

The concept of assent has been formalized. Since children cannot legally give permission for treatment or give "true informed consent" until they reach their 18th birthday, the concept of assent was supported. The AAP Committee on Bioethics (1995) and the National Cancer Institute (2020) state that children should participate in decision-making *commensurate with their development,* providing "assent" to care whenever reasonable. The term *assent* refers to a child's formal statements of contribution during decision-making. It is defined by the American Heritage College Dictionary as an "acceptance of and often belief in another's views, 'acquiescence,' 'consent,' or to 'agreement,' especially as a result of deliberation." The age of assent has been estimated as being about 12 (Foreman, 1999), although various institutions may have varying policies on the minimal age, including having children as young as 7 participate in family conferences or treatment decision-making.

According to the AAP Committee on Bioethics (1995), physicians should seek parental permission in most situations. They must focus on the goal of providing appropriate care and be prepared to seek legal intervention when parental refusal places the patient at clear and substantial risk. When the parents refuse "appropriate care," pediatricians should seek consultative assistance and use judicial determinations only in rare or unusual circumstances. Because only patients who have appropriate decisional capacity and legal empowerment can give their informed consent, assent of an underage child should be sought whenever appropriate and considered during treatment decisions.

PARENTAL PERMISSION

For physicians or primary providers to perform diagnostics, interventions, and medical services for a child, they must legally acquire parental permission. Permission is sought in two ways: the verbal agreement dictating permission from the parents after a discussion on the process, its risks and benefits, and alternatives available; and by a witnessed signature of the parent or legal guardian. There are times during administration of emergency care that verbal permission is sought, and a signature is acquired later, but this is not ideal. It is imperative, when both parties are able, to secure verbal permissions and a signature on a consent form to avoid the potential of litigation or confusion about the necessary medical interventions. Diagnostic evaluation, blood product transfusion, and minor or major procedures require parental (or legal guardian) permission by way of informed consent.

5 LEGAL IMPLICATIONS AND CONSENT

If parents are not willing to sign a consent form because of religious or cultural beliefs, state courts in the US have historically been willing to hold that religious convictions and beliefs, in and of themselves, are not a true defense to criminal liability for those families whose religious practices or cultural traditions exclude medical care (Greenawalk, 2008; Monopoli, 1991). In these cases, the physician may need to seek court interventions in the way of temporary guardianship to provide needed diagnostics and interventions. Full parental permission, support, and consent are ideal and smooth the process of providing healthcare to children, but they are not required to secure safe treatment for children.

CHAPTER 6

LEGAL PERSPECTIVES OF TREATMENT REFUSAL: REFUSAL DEFINED

An early definition of treatment refusal was given by Appelbaum and Roth (1983) as the "overt rejection by the patient, or his/her representative of medication, surgery, investigative procedures, or other components of hospital care recommended or ordered by the patient's physician" (p. 1296). According to the UK's National Health Service (2017), the right to refuse medical treatment should take place after full information is provided, "capacity" is present, and the patient's decision is made alone without pressure by family, friends, or any healthcare provider. Refusal of medically needed healthcare is no longer deemed an obscure phenomenon but rather has recently become the focus of literary attention.

When a parent refuses basic medical treatment deemed to be lifesaving, the healthcare team members may need to contact social workers, hospital officials, and possibly child protective agency representatives to petition juvenile or family court systems to obtain legally mandated temporary guardianship (Anderson, 1983; Linnard-Palmer & Kools, 2005; see Appendix D). Time should not be spent during the critical period of treatment decision-making attempting to change parental refusal for consent to treatment by asking the parents to give up their beliefs (Quintero, 1993).

According to Swan (1997), parents do not have a First Amendment right to abuse or neglect children. There is always the possibility of criminal liability when parents refuse medical treatment for their child based on religious or cultural beliefs. Swan (1997) states that only a minor fraction of cases of children dying because of treatment refusal based on religious doctrine have resulted in actual prosecution.

As discussed in a previous chapter, the three American constitutional bases for right to refuse treatment for competent adults—freedom from nonconsensual invasion, right of privacy, and the constitutional right to freedom of religion—do not apply to children who are of nonconsenting age or who are unemancipated minors. Governing bodies, such as individual state legislatures, create laws that protect the well-being of a child. These protective laws are under the umbrella of child abuse and neglect laws and are created to prevent human suffering, harm, and death due to parental acts of omission and commission.

According to research conducted by Asser and Swan (1998), parents who use faith healing rather than medical treatment may subject their children to unnecessary suffering and death from neglect, demonstrating that existing laws are insufficient in protecting children. Child fatalities in faith-healing sects were reviewed by Asser and Swan, and the probability of survival for each case was estimated based on survival rates expected of children who receive medical care for similar disorders. Their findings indicate that withholding medical treatment in favor of exclusive prayer leads to poorer health outcomes. Asser and Swan highly support laws that ensure safe, adequate, and thorough medical care for all children.

ROUTES OF LEGAL ACTIONS

Legal actions come in several forms. For instance, courts will allow, in general, the refusal of extraordinary care when the minor is either in a coma or considered to be terminally ill. In one such case, the Massachusetts Supreme Judicial Court allowed a "no code" status to be put in place for a child younger than 1 year old who was considered to be terminal. Another case involved a New Jersey father who was allowed by that state's Supreme Court to extubate an irreversibly comatose daughter (Rhodes & Miller, 1984). Courts do not intervene in situations where the families are offered unorthodox treatments or when the benefits do not clearly outweigh the risks. As described in the case of an 11-year-old with a severely deformed arm, the court refused to authorize amputation of the child's arm when the parents had refused the surgery and the physicians felt it was medically warranted.

Five reasons for courts to override a patient's right to refuse medical treatment have been noted within several US laws:

1. Preservation of life when the patient's condition is curable.
2. Protection of the patient's dependents, especially minor children.
3. Prevention of irrational self-destruction.

4. Preservation of ethical integrity of healthcare providers.
5. Protection of the public health and other interests.

In relation to minors, state laws generally focus on protecting the minor's welfare. In relation to children making consensual decisions about their healthcare, the UK's Children's Act of 1989 considers a 16-year-old to be capable of making their own treatment decision (Purssell, 1995). There have been instances where US physicians in pediatric oncology practice have granted autonomous treatment decisions to minors of 17 years of age, regardless of parental refusal or support of the child's cancer treatments. At the age of 17, children can proceed to become legally responsible for their healthcare treatment decision by applying for, and being granted, legal emancipation (Davis & Fang, 2020).

The adolescent patient under the age of 18 presents an increasing dilemma for healthcare professionals. Considered legally incompetent, by historical definition, adolescents "are legally unable to give informed consent for treatments, or to unilaterally refuse medically indicated treatments" (Lantos & Miles, 1989, p. 461). Current definitions confirm the importance of "respecting the developing autonomy of children, involving minors in decision-making" but determining a level of maturity required for "rational conversation-partners" to provide "decision-making competence" is challenging (Grootens-Wiegers et al., 2017, p. 1).

Two distinctly different situations can occur in the care of adolescents. They may align their religious or cultural beliefs with the parents and request withholding or limiting of certain medical treatments, or they may request to be treated against the parents' belief systems.

Six principles or concepts have been described concerning the dilemma around refusal or requests for medical treatment by an adolescent (see the nearby sidebar).

> ## Six Principles Concerning Adolescent Refusal of Medical Treatment
>
> 1. The physician's ethical obligation to act in a beneficent manner justifies emergency treatment.
>
> 2. The right to privacy in consideration of sexual or reproductive health leads to dilemmas in including parents' input.
>
> 3. The concept of a mature minor allowing the healthcare team to sidestep the legal presumption of incompetence and permitting treatment decision-making.
>
> 4. The right to religious freedom in decisions to refuse treatment is sometimes considered.
>
> 5. A multidisciplinary approach for determining decision-making competence is best (same-age children do not always demonstrate the same level of maturity).
>
> 6. Four child or adolescent capacities should be required: understanding, reasoning, decision-making, and communicating a treatment path choice. Yet, decision-making capacity (expressing a choice, abstract thinking) is necessary in treatment decisions for minors but is not sufficient for having decision-making competence (understanding consequences, risks, benefits, and having reasoning). Competence is a growing skill, not something that turns on and off during the developmental period.

All six of these guiding principles/concepts can leave medical professionals in a quandary. The obligation to act in emergency treatments, although logical and lifesaving, may indeed be acts against the belief systems of the family. If adolescents seek information or treatments for sexual/reproductive health issues while requesting privacy, and parents have made clear their cultural or religious beliefs to the care providers, conflicts may arise. If parents are highly verbalizing their wishes against medical treatment for a "mature minor" yet the minor is requesting to be treated, healthcare providers find themselves in a conflict of interest between parties. The right to religious freedom in decisions to refuse treatment may create a conflict for the healthcare provider when the adolescent may not fully comprehend the health risks. Solutions come from careful consideration of the wishes of all parties while applying the law.

As stated by Fink et al. (2010), less than 50% of adult patients or their surrogates truly comprehend consent for medical procedures; imagine the comprehension of a minor.

Legal doctrine pertaining to an adolescent refusing medical treatments continues to be unclear and may rest on the perception of the physician—i.e., the court may look to the physician(s) for guidance when endorsing treatment refusal. The two questions relating to decision-making by the courts that judges tend to ask physicians are:

1. Is there a medical need?
2. Is there a medically feasible response?

If both questions are answered affirmatively, judges may then provide the legal means required to administer treatments. Quality of life may not be considered for such decisions but rather the rule that if a lifesaving treatment is available, it should be undertaken (Canadian Paediatric Society, 2004).

From personal observations and conclusions drawn from interviews, it is apparent that the physician, and all members of the healthcare team, include the older school-age child and adolescent in treatment decision-making whenever possible. Harrison (2004) from the Canadian Paediatric Society's Bioethics Commitee offers a summary of principles (p. 1):

- Children, regardless of age, physical ability, or mental ability, have inherent value and should be protected and given medical treatment as needed.
- Pediatric healthcare professionals must keep minors' welfare in the forefront before family decisions that include treatment refusal.
- Interdisciplinary pediatric healthcare teams should keep family involved with treatment decisions whenever possible.
- When appropriate, a minor who has been deemed to have mature enough decision-making ability should be involved in treatment decisions.
- Interdisciplinary pediatric healthcare teams should use evidence-based information and present the information with veracity and sensitivity.
- Professionals should not allow their own viewpoints or values to influence or restrict medical treatment options presented to patients or their families.

HISTORICAL PERSPECTIVES OF TREATMENT REFUSAL

History provides a context in which to view the development of, or process of, how health sciences became what they are now. Considering that the first medical record was not developed for use in hospital and ambulatory settings until the early 20th century (Gillu, 2013), this clearly shows how far medicine and related fields have developed in a relatively short period of time. Now, the medical record is one of the most important tools to conduct research, prevent litigation, and track patient progress. Where were we before that time?

Treatment refusal within the science of pediatrics does not have a readily traceable history. Information became available after the first medical records were created and subsequently during the securing of child rights. No absolute way has been found to trace the accurate history of healthcare refusal scenarios or to document how influential church doctrines were historically developed. Nevertheless, historical perspectives of the development of influential court decisions around parental refusal or limitation of medical care were found in the literature from varied sources. These court decisions can be summarized in the following chronological list:

1878	Courts limited the right to certain religious practices where they impinged on the rights of others.
1891	The US Supreme Court recognized the right to refuse unwanted medical treatment for adults.
1903	Since the year 1903, American courts have held that the First Amendment to the Constitution for religious freedom does not give the right to withhold medical care from a child (People v. New York, Peirson).
1905	On February 20, 1905, the Supreme Court decided that the government has the power to protect citizens by forced vaccinations. In Jacobson v. Massachusetts, residents who refused to receive smallpox injections could be fined (Jacobson v. Massachusetts, 197 US 11, 1905).
1944	Supreme Court rulings stated, "The right to practice religion freely does not include the liberty to expose . . . a child . . . to ill health or death" (Prince v. Mass, 321 US 1944).

6 LEGAL PERSPECTIVES OF TREATMENT REFUSAL: REFUSAL DEFINED

1951   In all cases documented to this date, courts have ordered that children receive transfusions when medically indicated even against their parents' wishes to refuse. Courts may grant mandatory treatment orders over the phone within 15 minutes since most hospitals have 24-hour legal consults available (Fox, 1990).

1962   Courts upheld an adult patient's right to refuse blood on the grounds of protection of individual choice (even to the point of loss of human life).

1975   The US Department of Health, Education, and Welfare set forth regulations to implement the Child Abuse Prevention and Treatment Act of 1974, giving definitions and a requirement that a state include a prayer-treatment option.

1975   Family Court in New York deemed a parent who did not vaccinate their child as not being neglectful based on the parents' refusal of vaccines due to religious beliefs. The court determined that no official church membership was required (Parasidis & Opel, 2017).

1982   Baby Doe, born in 1982 in Bloomington, Indiana, with Down syndrome was born with a birth defect (duodenal atresia) requiring surgery. The baby's parents refused surgery. Hospital officials appointed a state guardian, but the court ruled in favor of the parents and against the surgery. The Indiana Supreme Court refused to appeal or even hear the case.

1983   The US Department of Health and Human Services removed the prayer-treatment exemption and defined child neglect to include denial of medical treatment.

1984   Amendment to the Child Abuse Prevention and Treatment Act occurred to include that all newborns must receive maximal life-prolonging treatment (Baby Doe regulation). Federal legislation was enacted to prevent neglect of handicapped infants.

1988   Neonatologists expressed concern to the US Supreme Court over Baby Doe regulation. The question of whether each case should go to court for review arose for intense scrutiny.

1989   Supreme Court reaffirms that "a competent person would have a constitutionally protected right to refuse lifesaving hydration and nutrition…thus causing death" (Cruzan by Cruzan v. Director, Missouri Department of Health, para. 4).

2013   The US District Court for the Southern District of West Virginia confirmed a verdict of child neglect for a mother who did not fully vaccinate her child, claiming that the physician's office refused care due to unpaid medical bills.

2018   A verdict was awarded to a parent whose child died of pneumococcal sepsis after refusing the pneumococcal vaccine for the infant. The claim was that during the refusal scenario, the parent said they were never told of the risk of death if the vaccine was not accepted (Scibilia, 2018).

Where are we now? The most recent position expressed by the American Academy of Pediatrics (AAP) was that exemptions should continue to be reevaluated and revoked as needed to ensure safe measures for ill children (AAP Policy Statement, 2013). Although the AAP's major concern is treating the child, the academy's position includes demonstrating sensitivity to and allowing for all voices to be heard.

CHAPTER 7

IN THE NAME OF RELIGION: HISTORICAL INFLUENCES TO LEGAL EXEMPTIONS

Religious exemptions from child abuse laws were first passed beginning in 1974 by all states as a reaction to a federal government mandate. US federal government authorities decided they would not allocate federal funds for any state for child protection programs unless religious exemptions were provided. Eleven states had exemptions in place by the end of 1974, and within 10 years, all states had an exemption in place. Some states (Arizona, Connecticut, Illinois, and Washington) met these federal requirements by providing religious exemptions to Christian Scientists only. One by one, states changed their exemptions over the years to allow greater ability to prosecute for withholding medical care as a form of child abuse, even though earlier the federal government promoted exemptions. At the time of this publication, all US states but Iowa and Ohio can prosecute for manslaughter when a child dies from parental treatment refusal based on religious doctrines (CHILD USA, n.d.).

As of 2018, 43 states exempt parents, at some level, for withholding medical care from their child based on the parents' religious beliefs (CHILD USA, 2020; Radcliffe, 2018). "In those states, if a parent refuses medical care for a child and opts instead for only spiritual treatment, the child won't be considered neglected under the law, even if they're harmed or die" (Radcliffe, 2018, para. 15). According to Dr. Rita Swan, as cited by Radcliffe (2018), "Faith-based medical neglect is the only kind of child abuse and neglect that's actually protected by law in many states" (para. 19). The extent of religious-based medical neglect cases in the US, or anywhere in the world, is unclear as the cases may not have been reported, records may not have been kept, and families may not have fully disclosed their situation to the authorities. Even with the presence of medical neglect in the auspices of religious beliefs, both local authorities and courts can step in and intervene by appointed guardianship that would lead to the medical treatment of a child.

In 2000, Swan reported that 41 states have exemptions for religious preference from child neglect or child abuse charges, while 31 states allow a religious defense from criminal charges. At that time, two states, Iowa and Ohio, still had religious exemptions from a prosecution of manslaughter, while Delaware and West Virginia continued to allow religious defenses for murder charges. One state, Arkansas, allowed for religious defenses against capital murder. As of 2016, all 50 states allow medical exemptions for certain patients, such as those who are immunocompromised or allergic to various vaccine components. Additionally, there are 30 states that allow exemptions for children whose parents cite religious reasons, and 18 states that make special accommodations for those expressing philosophical reasons. "States with a religious defense to child endangerment, criminal abuse or neglect, and cruelty to children include Alabama, Colorado, Delaware, Georgia, Idaho, Indiana, Iowa, Kansas, Louisiana, Maine, Minnesota, Missouri, Nevada, New Hampshire, New Jersey, New York, Ohio, Oklahoma, South Carolina, Tennessee, Texas, Utah, Virginia, West Virginia, and Wisconsin" (Swan, 2000, p. 8).

HISTORICAL INFLUENCES

The timeline goes as follows (Janofsky, 2001):

- Congress's 1974 directive required states receiving federal money for child abuse and prevention programs to have exemptions for parents who substituted prayer/healing for medical care.
- This directive was then rescinded in 1983, nine years later, as most states had already enacted religious exemptions.
- "Then in 1996, Congress seemed to reverse itself in the Child Abuse Prevention and Treatment Act, saying there was no federal requirement that a child must be provided any medical service or treatment against the religious beliefs of the parent or legal guardian" (Janofsky, 2001, p. 1).

In 2001, Congress reauthorized the federal Child Abuse Prevention and Treatment Act (CAPTA), requiring that states receiving federal money for programs against child abuse have laws requiring parents to provide needed healthcare services. However, CAPTA allows "statutory exemptions" for parents with religious objections.

Clearly, the history around this nation's government's commitment to protect children is confusing and may have been highly influenced by organized religions lobbying for their protection against prosecution. Swan (2000, p. 9) asks a succinct question:

> Why, in the twenty-first century, is this situation allowed to continue? It may be because the United States remains reluctant to fully acknowledge children as right-bearing persons. The public and its lawmakers aren't ready to give children a constitutional right to health care. While states do require parents to provide their children with the necessities of life, they don't always require that children receive adequate health care. And every state, at one time or another, has passed laws allowing parents to withhold on religious grounds some forms of medical treatment. Religious exemption laws create two classes of children. One is entitled to preventive, diagnostic and therapeutic health care because their parents have a legal duty to provide it. The other—those in faith-healing sects—have no right to immunizations, prophylactic eye drops, health screenings and, depending on the reach of the religious defense in the criminal code, no right to medical care for illnesses unless and until a state agency becomes aware of their needs and obtains care by court order.

Some states continue to have religious exemptions for immunizations and metabolic testing for newborns. Delaware, Illinois, Kansas, Maine, Massachusetts, New Jersey, and Rhode Island allow exemptions for testing for lead levels in a child's blood. California, Colorado, Massachusetts, Michigan, Minnesota, and Ohio have statutes that allow students with religious objectives to be excused from studying about human diseases. Other medical exemptions based on religious beliefs include refusal of eye drops for newborns, tuberculosis testing, school health screenings, hearing screenings for newborns, vitamin K shots for newborns to prevent bleeding disorders, and even bicycle helmets (CHILD USA, 2020; Kraszewski et al., 2006).

7 IN THE NAME OF RELIGION

The national office of the American Civil Liberties Union made a statement in regard to the presence of religious exemptions (www.masskids.org, 2021, para 5):

> Children have rights too, and parents have certain rights which end when they intrude too far into a child's right to live ... the parent's right to bring up the child in the way the parent thinks best—an important right—ends at the point which the parents' actions endanger the lives of kids ... there cannot be in our view a religious exemption no matter how sincere a parent's belief.

In 1983, the US Department of Health and Human Services (DHHS) no longer mandated that states include exemptions for religious doctrines that influence healthcare decisions for children. Rather, the DHHS requires states to provide medical treatment in their definitions of child neglect (Swan, 1997). In fact, in 1996, Congress added to the Child Abuse Prevention and Treatment Act amendments that require parents to provide needed medical services to a child, even against their religious or cultural beliefs, and imposed a moratorium on DHHS requiring changes in revoking religious exemptions laws (Swan, 1997).

Historically, many states have exemptions to their child abuse and neglect laws for spiritual (or religious) treatment. These exemptions do not mean that the courts will not intervene on behalf of the child, especially when the child is in a life-threatening situation. This troublesome conflict within the legal system continues to be addressed in our courts. The states' authority to act as a guardian for those children who are unable to care for themselves continues to be deeply entrenched in the law (Neely, 1998; Swan, 2020b).

Historical examples of legal exemptions to laws based on beliefs are interesting. Some states exempt children from having to wear bicycle helmets if the parents' belief system objects. Other states allow parents not to immunize their children against childhood infectious diseases (when there is no current epidemic of those diseases) and therefore, based on beliefs, may send their children to public school without immunizations.

According to Swan (n.d., CHILD's public policy achievements):

> Since 1990, Arizona, Colorado, Delaware, Hawaii, Maryland, Massachusetts, Minnesota, North Carolina, Rhode Island, Oregon, South Dakota, and Tennessee have repealed some or all religious exemptions from a duty to provide medical care for a sick child. CHILD gave extensive support to repeal bills in several of those states and has blocked the Christian Science church from getting more religious exemptions enacted in some states. Presentations by CHILD members to the American Academy of Pediatrics, American Medical Association, National Child Abuse Coalition, National Committee for the Prevention of Child Abuse (now Prevent Child Abuse America), U.S. Advisory Board on Child Abuse and Neglect, National District Attorneys Association, United Methodist Church, and the National Association of Medical Examiners contributed to those organizations' adoption of policy statements against religious exemptions.

Organized religious groups can be quite influential on the writing and passing of state law. Much work lies ahead to ensure that there will not be two classes of children—those who receive fair access to and follow-through of healthcare and those whose parents are protected in withholding health teaching, health screening, preventive health measures, medical treatments, and lifesaving measures.

In conclusion, Dwyer (1996), a lawyer, writes in his article about children of religious objectors:

> When children whose parents fail, for religious reasons, to secure or consent to necessary medical care for them to

come to the attention of state officials, courts have some authority to order medical treatment over the parents' objections. A substantial amount of litigation and commentary has surrounded the question of when a court order is appropriate. Courts have uniformly found it appropriate to order medical treatment for a child, over parents' objection that doing so violates their First Amendment right to the free exercise of religion, when treatment is necessary to prevent the child from dying. Most courts have held that intervention is also appropriate when necessary to prevent 'grievous harm' to a child, which one state court defined as 'a significant impairment of vital physical or mental functions, protracted disability, permanent disfigurement, or similar defects or infirmities.' (pp. 1355–1356)

CLERGY RESPONSIBILITY AND THE LAW

Most churches have a leadership group responsible for the oversight of the structure and function of the organization. In some religious organizations, clergy are responsible for finances and daily operations. In others, clergy are a separate constituent whose sole responsibility is to teach, model, and apply church doctrine, leaving the day-to-day responsibility of church function to a church governing body. Whatever the structure, clergy can be seen as highly influential to the church community in the application of religious doctrine. Most states see this position as one of power and influence and therefore may hold the clergy member responsible for the outcomes of religious doctrine application. Parents, on the other hand, may deviate from their church's beliefs, doctrines, or teachings and proceed on their own faith path.

AGAINST MEDICAL ADVICE

The legal responsibility of the leaders of the churches whose doctrines and teachings influence or affect health-related decisions is an influencing factor in medical treatment refusal. Great legal commentary exists as to the level of legal responsibility the clergy should have when a child is harmed or dies from a delay or abstinence of traditional medical treatment based on religious doctrine. Discussions can be found in the literature concerning "clergy malpractice." According to Dodes (1987), a "typical clergy malpractice action alleges conduct such as improper pastoral counseling, intentional infliction of emotional distress, inadequate teaching or intentional interference with contractual relations, and the plaintiffs sue as representatives of the injured or deceased child" (p. 166).

As discussed in the Dodes (1987) article, on the other hand, the First Amendment to the US Constitution provides that Congress will not make laws that prohibit the free practice of one's religion. This demonstrates that there is no complete separation of church and state.

In actions alleging church negligence, the plaintiffs are often unable to proceed with their litigation because of the constitutionally protected nature of church conduct under US federal and individual state constitutions. Although the controversy would be justifiable if the defendants were private individuals, churches have been absolved from civil litigation by virtue of the doctrine of separation of church and state. "Policy which supports the judicial rule of preventing adjudication of a negligence action against a religious organization should not serve to insulate faith healers from liability by preventing legal recourse to families of children being sacrificed in the name of religion" (Dodes, 1987, pp. 166–168). It is important to emphasize that many religious institutions and members believe in prayer for healing. However, conflict can arise when certain groups do not accept modern Western medical treatment.

What is interesting to note is that *belief* and *conduct* are seen as two distinctly different words. Religious *belief* affecting children may be exempt from the First Amendment protection, whereas religious *conduct* (also known as *practices*) may not be. If a church is immune from civil liability, it may be because the medical treatment refusal for a child was considered to be *secular conduct,* which can be regulated by law, versus *secular beliefs*, which cannot (Cornell Law School, 2020; Dodes, 1987).

LEGAL EXEMPTIONS TO SPECIFIC TYPES OF HEALTHCARE/ TREATMENTS

In the US, some states have kept legislation in place to allow exemptions from routine health screening, immunizations, and other specific health-related childhood interventions.

According to CHILD USA (2020), exemptions from preventive and diagnostic measures continue to exist, even though these measures are widely known to prevent childhood diseases, injuries, and illnesses. For example, some states continue to have exemptions for newborn metabolic testing. These tests detect the presence of an actual or potential disease in the neonate for which there may be interventions to prevent illness, blindness, mental retardation, or even death.

A common prevention for severe disease, and sometimes blindness, in newborns is the administration of antimicrobial eye drops in all newborns. Chlamydia and gonorrhea are two of the microbial infections that can be easily prevented by the routine instillation of eye drops for all neonates (CDC, 2019a). Colorado, Iowa, Michigan, and Minnesota all have religious exemptions for families to refuse eye drops for their neonates based on religious beliefs. According to CHILD USA (2021), most states have laws allowing religious exemptions to health screenings of children. Additional exemptions can be found in Table 7.1.

Table 7.1 Religious Exemption Laws by State

Religious Exemption	States
Routine health screening offered as preventative healthcare in public schools	California, Colorado, Michigan, Minnesota, and Ohio (CHILD USA, 2020; Swan, 2000, p. 7)
Hearing tests for newborns	California, Connecticut, New Jersey, and West Virginia (CHILD USA, 2020; Swan, 2000, p. 7)
Studying about disease in school	California, Colorado, Massachusetts, Michigan, Minnesota, and Ohio (CHILD USA, 2020; Swan, 2000, p. 7)
Routine screening of children for lead poisoning	Illinois, Iowa, Louisiana, Maryland, Ohio, Rhode Island, Virginia, and West Virginia (Networkforphl.org, 2019)
Refusal of eye drops for neonates	Colorado, Iowa, Michigan, and Minnesota (CHILD USA, 2020; Swan, 2000, p. 7; wvlegislature.gov (2018)
Refusal of intramuscular vitamin K in neonates	Tennessee: In 2013, there were four cases of late onset vitamin K deficiency bleeding due to parental refusal of IM vitamin K for their newborns. In all four cases, the refusal was due to information the parents found on the internet giving them concerns over synthetic or toxic ingredients and the belief that it would be "unnatural." These parents were unaware of the risk of intracranial bleeding or death that could arise because of their vitamin K refusal (Monroe et al., 2018).

| Refusal of school immunization requirements | At the time of this writing, 45 states and Washington, DC grant religious exemptions for religious objections to immunizations. Colorado, for instance, requires an online education module to be submitted for exemptions (NCSL.org, 2021). |

Lead Poisoning: A Silent Disorder

Lead poisoning is often a silent disorder where a child's blood levels of lead slowly rise without gross detectable signs. When a child's level reaches a certain point, many body systems can be affected, and it can lead to massive neurological damage, seizures, coma, and death. Lead poisoning continues to plague this nation. Recent events in Flint, Michigan are a perfect example. Contaminated water from the Flint River elevated lead levels by threefold in community members, leading to 18 months of significant health issues (NRDC.org). Lead poisoning is also highly influenced by the influx of immigrants whose homelands may have unrestricted lead substances (gasoline, construction paint, ceramic paints, and industrial exposures) present in the soil, food, and cookware. Children who are not screened but are at risk may suffer several disorders and symptoms including anemia, nausea, neurological symptoms such as developmental delays, learning difficulties, and failure to thrive (Mayoclinic.org, 2019).

CHAPTER 8

ADULT MEDICAL TREATMENT REFUSALS, LIMITATIONS, AND DELAYS

There are many studies investigating the contributing factors related to hospital discharges AMA. There is much interest in this subject because AMA discharges result in higher healthcare costs, increased readmission rates, and higher mortality (Choi et al., 2011; Kraut et al., 2013; Lee et al., 2016). One retrospective analysis of 1,770,570 trauma patients admitted during the years 2013 to 2015 found that 24,191 patients (1.4%) had left AMA (Haines et al., 2019). More specifically, a total of 19,450 patients left AMA from the hospital, and 4,741 left AMA from the ED. Here are some interesting findings. According to Haines et al. (2019):

- Uninsured patients were almost three times more likely to leave AMA than privately insured patients.
- Medicaid patients were 2.5 times more likely to leave AMA than privately insured patients.
- African American patients were more likely than Caucasian patients to leave AMA.
- Use of alcohol or illicit drugs resulted in an increased likelihood of leaving AMA.

In addition to the above-noted characteristics, previous research studies have indicated that being homeless, being male, having left AMA before, or having a history of several different co-morbidities (e.g., psychiatric illness, hepatitis C, HIV) are all associated with higher rates of leaving AMA (Lee et al., 2016; Menendez et al., 2015; Spooner et al., 2017).

Suggested Interventions to Decrease AMA Discharges

Perform early identification of uninsured patients, vulnerable populations (e.g., homeless), patients who might be experiencing racial discrimination, patients with substance abuse issues, patients with serious comorbid conditions, patients with a history of mental illness, and patients with a prior history of leaving AMA. Specifically:

- These high-risk patients should receive closer attention from the moment they are admitted.
- Care should be taken to actively engage them in their treatment plan.

> - Their caregivers should be culturally appropriate and/or culturally sensitive.
> - Strategies for enhanced communication should be developed.
> - Consultation with a therapist or other trained specialized individuals should be offered as appropriate.
> - Discharge AMA should be reframed more positively and viewed as an opportunity for active listening, compassion, patient engagement, and shared decision-making.

MEDICATION NONADHERENCE

While the acute care setting studies AMA discharges, the outpatient and/or primary care literature tends to focus more upon medication nonadherence. It has been estimated that approximately 40% to 80% of patients are nonadherent to their prescribed medication regimes—especially those with chronic conditions (Cohen et al., 2012). Obviously, this is a serious issue, as medication adherence is crucial for successfully attaining one's clinical treatment goals. Furthermore, it has been estimated that approximately 30% of medicine-related hospital admissions occur because of medication nonadherence (Osterberg & Blaschke, 2005). In fact, "Medication nonadherence for diabetes, heart failure, hyperlipidemia, and hypertension result in billions of Medicare FFS [fee-for-service] expenditures, millions in hospital days, and thousands of ED visits that could have been avoided" (Lloyd et al., 2019, p. 218).

To solve issues related to medication nonadherence, it is first necessary to understand the characteristics of the people who do not comply with their treatment plan. Male gender; being African American, Hispanic, or another cultural minority; being single; and a high frequency of medication doses per day were all associated with nonadherence (Davidson, Lam, & Sokn, 2019). Somewhat counterintuitively, older age is associated with *increased* medication compliance. One explanation theorized by Cohen et al. (2012) is that older adults have more interactions with the healthcare system and a higher level of experience with managing medications. However, a different study based on a 2013–2015 National Health Interview Survey found that older adults who were experiencing food insecurity or who were threatened by hunger were significantly more likely to engage in cost-related medication nonadherence (CRN; Blewett et al., 2016). CRN can include delaying filling a prescription, skipping medications, or taking smaller doses to save money (Srinivasan & Pooler, 2018). For older adults who are being nonadherent to their prescribed medications due to lack of money, it is very important to enroll them in SNAP (state nutrition assistance programs) and any other benefit programs for which they may be eligible. A study by Srinivasan and Pooler (2018) found that SNAP may help older adults better afford their medications by reducing out of pocket expenses for food. Unfortunately, only 4 in 10 eligible adults aged 60 years and older participate in SNAP (Farson & Cunnynham, 2016). Therefore, every eligible older adult should be assisted in removing and/or addressing any perceived barriers in accessing this important program.

COMMUNICATION TECHNIQUES FOR ADULT REFUSALS, LIMITATIONS, AND DELAYS

In recent years, motivational interviewing has increasingly been utilized in primary care practice. This technique was initially conceived by William R. Miller in 1983 (Rubak et al., 2005) to assist patients who were struggling with alcoholism. Later, Stephen Rollnick joined Miller, and together they developed the theory into a more detailed clinical process with the capacity to be useful in many different contexts, including immunization hesitancy and other treatment refusals, limitations, and delays. Motivational interviewing has been "particularly useful for clients who are reluctant to change or who are ambivalent about changing their behavior" (Rubak et al., 2005, p. 305). It is a patient-centered approach that assists the person in identifying, understanding, and overcoming their own barriers to change. It can help to resolve ambivalence and it can motivate through questioning and advice.

Characteristics of Motivational Interviewing

- Motivational interviewing relies upon identifying and mobilizing the client's intrinsic values and goals to stimulate behavior change.
- Motivation to change is elicited from the client and not imposed from without.
- Motivational interviewing is designed to elicit, clarify, and resolve ambivalence and to perceive benefits and costs associated with it.
- Readiness to change is not a client trait but a fluctuating product of interpersonal interaction.
- Resistance and denial are often a signal to modify motivational strategies.
- Eliciting and reinforcing the client's belief in ability to carry out and succeed in achieving a specific goal is essential.
- The therapeutic relationship is a partnership with respect to client autonomy.
- Motivational interviewing is both a set of techniques and a counseling style.
- Motivational interviewing is directive and client-centered counseling, understanding, and eliciting behavior change.

(Miller & Rollnick, 2013)

According to a meta-analysis of randomized controlled trials using motivational interviewing as the intervention, motivational interviewing was found to be more effective than traditional advice giving. Even one brief encounter of just 15 minutes showed an effect when using motivational interviewing; however, more than one encounter with the patient was ideal (Rubak et al., 2004). It should be emphasized that motivational interviewing is particularly applicable to conditions that are amenable to behavior change related to lifestyle choices such as exercise, weight control, smoking cessation, diabetes, asthma control, medication adherence, etc.

THE CONFUSED MIND ALWAYS SAYS, "NO!"

"The confused mind always says 'No'" is a well-known maxim from marketing. Nonetheless, it has plenty of potential for application to healthcare. These authors remember observing a nursing student presentation on the topic of asthma prepared for a group of young schoolchildren. The nursing students had worked hard on their presentation, and they meant well, but they were using words such as *bronchiole* and *alveoli*, and it was obvious that these terms were going right over the heads of their 2nd-grade audience. Obviously, people cannot be expected to follow a treatment plan that they cannot understand, no matter what their age is.

Accordingly, one of the first considerations when working with any patient, group, or target population should be to consider their health literacy level. To address the problem of health literacy, the CDC (2019c) has put together five talking points about health literacy that can be adapted to advocate for promotion of health literacy (see the nearby sidebar).

8 ADULT MEDICAL TREATMENT REFUSALS, LIMITATIONS, AND DELAYS

Common Reasons Adult Patients Say "No!" to Their Treatment Plan

- They are confused by being given too many treatment options.
- The elements of their treatment plan are not delivered in a structured way that makes sense to them.
- The presentation of the treatment plan is too rushed.
- They are not given the chance to ask questions, or they are scared to ask questions because of fear of appearing ignorant.
- There is a language barrier, and understanding the communication is difficult.
- They feel overwhelmed, anxious, or self-conscious and are unable to absorb the details.
- Technical jargon and terms they do not understand are used.
- They do not understand the value of their treatment plan and/or they have misconceptions about it.

The CDC's Five Talking Points on Health Literacy

You are a health literacy ambassador. It is up to you to make sure your colleagues, staff, leadership, and community are aware of the issues. Whether to review for yourself, present to others, or convince your leadership, the following resources may help you talk about health literacy.

These five brief talking points may be helpful if you need to tell someone quickly what health literacy is and why it is important (CDC, 2019c). Add in talking points relevant to your organization.

1. Nine out of 10 adults struggle to understand and use health information when it is unfamiliar, complex, or jargon-filled.

2. Limited health literacy costs the healthcare system money and results in higher than necessary morbidity and mortality.

3. Health literacy can be improved if we practice clear communication strategies and techniques.

4. Clear communication means using familiar concepts, words, numbers, and images presented in ways that make sense to the people who need the information.

5. Testing information with the audience before it is released and asking for feedback are the best ways to know if we are communicating clearly. We need to test and ask for feedback every time information is released to the general public.

Although there are tools for assessing health literacy, the current recommendation is to use *universal health literacy precautions*, which refers to providing all patients with information (both oral and written) that is understandable and easily accessible to persons across all education levels.

HEALTH BELIEF MODEL

The Health Belief Model (HBM) is a widely applied framework that can clarify health behavior. This model is also useful in that it may prompt the nurse to carefully consider what motivates people to change. According to Stanhope and Lancaster (2016), the HBM has six components (pp. 366–367):

1) Perceived susceptibility ("Will something happen to me?")

2) Perceived severity ("If something does happen to me, will it be a big problem?")

3) Perceived benefits ("If I do what is suggested, will it really help me?")

4) Perceived barriers ("Assuming I do what is suggested, will there be barriers that will be unpleasant, costly, and so forth?")

5) Cues to action ("What might motivate me to actually do something?")

6) Self-efficacy ("Can I really do this?")

Unfortunately, despite a large body of research supporting the influence of HBM variables on health behavior, there is still quite a bit of ambiguity concerning which variables are most important and how the variables interact within the model. Still, the HBM can help nurses understand: 1) how people involved feel about the health problem, 2) whether they think the problem is serious, 3) whether they think that action on their part will make a difference, and 4) whether they think they can both manage the barriers and actually perform the action (Edberg, 2013; Stanhope & Lancaster, 2016).

GLOBAL PERSPECTIVES ON HEALTH, ILLNESS, AND TREATMENT

The concepts of health and disease differ among Western and non-Western cultures, and cultural beliefs about what does or does not constitute appropriate treatment is greatly influenced by a person's cultural background and environment. Indeed, how we communicate about our illness, whom we consult when we require care, how long we remain in care, and whether we follow the treatment plan are greatly affected by our cultural beliefs.

The biomedical model that is predominant in Western culture takes the view that each disease has a specific cause and specific features that are universal throughout the world. It is grounded in science, and one of its core elements is germ theory, which emerged in the 19th century based on research done by Louis Pasteur in the 1850s, whose work was later expanded on by Robert Koch in the 1890s (Ibeneme et al., 2017). However, in non-Western cultures, the sociocultural model predominates. In this model, illness either arises from the actions of a malevolent being, the supernatural, or from an imbalance in the natural or social environment. For example, in some Hispanic and Asian cultures, illness is thought to be an imbalance between hot and cold humors. Hot conditions should be treated with cold therapies and vice versa (Ibeneme et al., 2017). And in some Latinx cultures, hypertension is considered a hot condition and, as such, should be managed with a cold treatment. Diabetes and peptic ulcer disease are two additional examples of hot conditions. Some cold conditions are cancer, colic, headache, and pneumonia (Juckett, 2005). In Ayurvedic medicine (practiced in certain parts of India), many foods are thought to have hot or cool qualities. "Garam or hot foods include eggs, meat, milk, dahl, honey, and sugar. Tonda or cold foods include fruit, yogurt, acid buttermilk, rice, and water" (Ibeneme et al., 2017, p. 15). The idea is that the right foods can restore the proper balance and help to treat or avert illness. It is not only foods that are ascribed hot or cold designations. Illnesses can be categorized as hot or cold as well. Even in the westernized United States, the idea of "food-as-medicine" has gained a lot of traction (Gorn, 2017). Food as medicine is making inroads as physicians and medical institutions make food a formal part of treatment (by prescribing nutritional changes), rather than relying solely on medications. In Southern California, Loma Linda University Health (n.d.-b) is offering specialized training for its resident physicians in lifestyle medicine—that's a formal subspecialty in using food to treat disease.

INDIVIDUAL WORLDVIEW AND ITS IMPACT ON HEALTHCARE DECISIONS

A person's worldview can also have profound healthcare implications. For example, people with a very fatalistic worldview may refuse to treat their chronic condition because they feel that treatment will not make any difference, as the outcome is already predetermined. Similarly, people who believe that their diabetes is "God's will" may refuse treatment because it would be wrong to resist the will of God. Immigrants to Western societies do not necessarily change their beliefs about what constitutes appropriate treatment for an illness. It is even possible that some may be in transition between two different paradigms and can hold conflicting beliefs concurrently. It has been estimated that up to 75% of all self-recognized episodes of sickness are managed outside the formal healthcare system (Ibeneme et al., 2017). The individual usually tries to treat herself first (sometimes using home remedies). Next, advice is sought from family or extended family. If the illness persists, a traditional healer from the person's own culture might be consulted. Finally, the person might access the conventional Western medical system, but the person may lose confidence in her clinician if she doesn't receive care that is culturally congruent with her beliefs. Therefore, the importance of cultural competence among nurses and other healthcare providers cannot be overemphasized. Efforts to provide culturally competent care can enrich the nurse-patient relationship and improve treatment adherence. A study by Hooper et al. (2018, p. 9) found that "patients who perceive their providers to be culturally competent are more likely to adhere to treatment." Similarly, patients who do not feel welcome in the healthcare environment or who do not feel their provider cares enough about them are less likely to follow their treatment plan (Hooper et al., 2018).

A cross-cultural interview should always be done when caring for a new patient (see the nearby sidebar). A good cross-cultural interview can clarify patient goals and reveal conceptual differences that need to be addressed in the treatment plan to foster better patient adherence, increased patient satisfaction, and improved therapeutic outcomes.

AVOIDANT HEALTH-SEEKING BEHAVIORS IN THE BLACK COMMUNITY

By Danielle EK Perkins, PhD, RN

The long history of medical abuses against the Black community continues to contribute to ongoing hesitance and even avoidant health-seeking behaviors. While the Tuskegee experiment seems to be the most readily invoked example of mistreatment, the historical context of early slave involvement in torturous medical experimentation should not be overlooked (Gamble, 1997). In addition, the current day-to-day experiences of Black people in the American healthcare system often unfortunately and negatively reinforce these beliefs and behaviors. The collective psyche of distrust by a large proportion of

Black people is further validated by current and startling quantitative evidence, in the form of health disparities.

Health disparities experienced by Black communities serve as evidence of healthcare system failures to provide equitable and efficacious assessment, diagnosis, treatment, and support. Maternal mortality for Black women is unacceptably high, even though most pregnancy-related deaths are preventable. Non-Hispanic Black women experience a pregnancy-related mortality ratio that is 3.2 times higher than that of white women (Centers for Disease Control and Prevention, 2019b). Even solidly middle-class, educated, and insured Black men and women have worse health outcomes than Whites with lower socioeconomic standing. For example, the pregnancy-related mortality rate for Black women with a college degree was 5.2 times higher than among white women with a high school diploma (American Heart Association, 2019). Unfortunately, similar disparities in cancer, heart disease, and stroke persist despite increasing levels of education for African Americans (Hamilton, 2017).

As alluded to early in this text, Black people are at a greater risk of leaving AMA. Black race is further compounded with intersections of low socioeconomic status, absence of health insurance, and less education—all of which contribute to poor health outcomes in some Black communities (Noonan et al., 2016). However, the present status of health inequality and disparities has a lineage rooted in slavery and early medical experimentation on Black bodies. Many of the advances in healthcare that patients benefit from today are a result of trauma inflicted upon Black women and men in the 1800s (Gamble, 1997; Washington, 2006). In fact, Dr. Marion J. Simms, often referred to as the father of gynecology, perfected procedures for surgical treatment of vesicovaginal and rectovaginal fistulas on slave women. He conducted his painful experiments without anesthesia because of the belief that Black women did not experience pain (Washington, 2006). Despite the racist paradigm for this misconception about Black people, it has continued to persist (University of Virginia, 2020).

These early abuses set the stage for ongoing violations and mistreatment of Black people in the American healthcare system. As recently as 1993, the New York State Psychiatric Institute conducted experiments exclusively on 34 Black and Hispanic boys between the ages of 6–10 without the full informed consent of their parents (Hilts, 1998). Hilts (1998) published a story in *The New York Times* detailing the study, reporting that the boys "were given intravenous doses of fenfluramine to test a theory that violent or criminal behavior may be predicted by levels of certain brain chemicals" (p. 3). While the implications of the Tuskegee experiment continue to haunt a generation of Black men and women, more recent violations that may not have been as publicized in the mainstream reside in the minds of Black people—in the Northeast and South at the very least.

Widespread distrust of non-minority medical providers and the association of healthcare institutions with maltreatment result in hesitance, resistance, or avoidant health-seeking behaviors for many Black people (Gamble, 1997). Unfortunately, subconscious biases and racist and discriminatory beliefs and behaviors continue to perpetuate much of the disparity in healthcare and the distrust in the Black community.

Notably, there are other dynamics that contribute to hesitation and avoidant health-seeking behaviors. The unique role that religion plays in health-maintenance behaviors of Black people has been found to be both health-protective and threatening (Hotz, 2015). The sometimes-insidious fatalism that underpins faith in the Black community should be considered for its negative impact on advantageous health-seeking and therapeutic-adherent behaviors. For example, among a sample of ethnically diverse adults and children diagnosed with asthma, belief in God was more strongly associated with low medication adherence among African Americans in the sample compared to whites (Ahmedani et al., 2013). Absolute belief in the power of prayer and its ability to cure illnesses and heal injuries is a lingering paradigm born out of an ongoing and yet historical memory of betrayal by the healthcare system (Hotz, 2015). The expression

"I don't claim that" is a form of resistance sometimes incantated by marginalized elder Black women in the church in response to a serious diagnosis such as cancer or diabetes (Hotz, 2015). "I don't claim that" is representative of a psychological refusal of permission that would allow illness to enter the body (Hotz, 2015). Such beliefs may be indicative of denial and result in a lack of treatment seeking or failure to adhere to a therapeutic regimen. In fact, some religious leaders in the Black community suggest that seeking healthcare represents a lack of faith (Hotz, 2015). It is difficult to quantify the extent to which these beliefs negatively impact the health and health outcomes of Black people, as more research is needed to fully understand this phenomenon.

Building upon an understanding of the significance of the Black church and its impact on health, it is important to recognize the essential role of Black clergy serving as first-line mental healthcare providers for Black people in their communities. Compared to other ethnic minorities, Blacks are less likely to seek counseling from mental health professionals (Avent et al., 2015). However, given the disparate rates of mental illness among Black people, this can be quite problematic (Noonan et al., 2016). Barriers to mental healthcare–seeking behaviors are primarily associated with the cultural stigma of mental illness, though distrust of providers and a lack of providers of color are also contributing factors (Avent et al., 2015). Given the varying educational background, knowledge of mental health and illness, and beliefs and messaging by Black faith leaders, it is unknown to what extent these factors negatively impact Black mental health help-seeking behaviors.

The influences and historical contexts that may often explain the interactions between the Black community and the US healthcare system are unique. There is no one-size-fits-all approach for understanding behaviors that would seem counterproductive to health protection. Rather, a clinician who has some contextual understanding and genuine and intrinsically motivated curiosity during the patient interview and assessment provides the best possible environment for success in achieving mutually determined goals for the patient's individual plan of care.

> ### Suggested Questions to Include in a Cross-Cultural Interview
>
> 1. What do you call the illness?
> 2. What do you think has caused the illness?
> 3. Why do you think the illness started when it did?
> 4. What problems do you think the illness causes? How does it work?
> 5. How severe is the illness? Will it have a long or short course?
> 6. What kind of treatment is necessary? What are the most important results you hope to receive from this treatment?
> 7. What are the main problems this illness has caused you?
> 8. What do you fear most about the illness?
>
> Note: Adapted from Juckett (2005)

BELIEF IN ALTERNATIVE THERAPIES

In the last two decades, there has been a large surge of interest in complementary and alternative therapy in the US. These include homeopathy, osteopathy, naturopathy, hypnosis, acupuncture, and various mind-body treatment modalities such as meditation, biofeedback, hypnosis, yoga, tai chi, and qi gong. In 2002, the CDC performed a study to estimate how many US adults use complementary and alternative medicine (CAM). Accordingly, the National Center

8 ADULT MEDICAL TREATMENT REFUSALS, LIMITATIONS, AND DELAYS

for Health Statistics (NCHS) collected data from 31,044 surveys of adults age 18 and over. They found that 62% of adults had used some form of CAM during the previous 12 months when prayer was included. When prayer was excluded from the definition of CAM, 36% of adults had used some form of CAM—still a significant number. NCHS also found that only 11.8% of adults sought care from a licensed or certified CAM practitioner. This indicates that many people who use CAM self-prescribe and/or self-medicate. In addition, NCHS found that many CAM users do not inform their healthcare providers about their use of herbal supplements, megavitamins, and/or other products (Barnes et al., 2004). According to a study by the IOM Committee on the Use of Complementary and Alternative Medicine (2005), among the respondents who reported their reasons for nondisclosure, common reasons were:

- "It wasn't important for the doctor to know" (61%)
- "The doctor never asked" (60%)
- "It was none of the doctor's business" (31%)
- "The doctor would not understand" (20%)

Fewer respondents (14%) thought that their doctor would disapprove of or discourage CAM use, and just 2% thought that the doctor might not continue as their provider if the doctor knew that the patient had received some sort of CAM therapy (IOM, 2005). Nondisclosure of anything a patient is taking—whether it is an herbal remedy, a megavitamin, or some other substance (prescribed or over the counter)—could have potentially serious consequences. However, even when patients do inform their conventional healthcare providers what they are taking, the clinician may not be acquainted with the product and may not be aware of the interactions and other ramifications of the patient's CAM use. According to the NCHS 2002 report, the reasons adults use CAM were as follows:

- They believed that CAM combined with conventional medical treatments would help (54.9%).

- They thought it would be interesting to try (50.1%).
- A medical professional suggested they try it (26%).
- They believed conventional medical treatments would not help (28%).
- They felt conventional medicine was too expensive (13%).

According to the NCHS study, some of the characteristics of CAM users are as follows (Barnes et al., 2004):

- Men were not as likely to use CAM as women. The largest difference was seen in the use of mind-body therapies, including prayer for health-related reasons.
- Older adults were more likely to utilize CAM than younger adults (if prayer was included). If prayer was not included, there was a U-shaped curve with the youngest and the oldest groups using CAM the least.
- 63.3% of Black adults were likely to use mind-body therapies (including prayer) compared to 50.1% of White adults and 48.1% of Asians.
- Poor adults were more likely to use CAM than wealthier adults.
- Persons with more education were more likely to use CAM than people who were less educated.
- A high number of people use CAM to treat musculoskeletal conditions and/or other conditions associated with chronic pain.

The most often-mentioned CAM therapies were chiropractic care, acupuncture, herbal medicine, hypnosis, massage therapy, relaxation techniques, biofeedback, homeopathic treatment, chelation therapy, energy therapies, qi gong, tai chi, yoga, high-dose vitamins, and spirituality/prayer for health purposes (Barnes et al., 2004). Other findings in the NCHS report indicated that Black and Asian adults were substantial users of CAM at 71.3% and 61.7%, respectively. This was new information at the time this report was published. Even more surprising was the finding that 27.7% of the people who use CAM believe that conventional medicine will not help their healthcare problem (Barnes et al., 2004).

ADULT VACCINE REFUSAL AND HESITANCY

Patient fears related to vaccines are well-publicized in the media. Soon after the COVID-19 pandemic began, there were a flurry of articles in the lay press replete with anti-vaccinators vowing to refuse any coronavirus vaccines that might be produced. According to the National Public Health Information Coalition, "Anti-vaxxers are terrified the government will 'enforce' a vaccine for coronavirus" (NPHIC, 2020, p. 1). On May 29, 2020, the British newspaper *The Guardian* published an article stating: "In early May, a survey by two academics found that 23% of Americans would not be willing to get vaccinated against COVID-19" (Gabbatt, 2020, para. 4). In a separate poll conducted January 24–26, 2020, by Morning Consult, 18% of people surveyed said they would not get vaccinated, and another 44% were unsure. However, in a subsequent poll conducted by Morning Consult from February 28 to March 1, 2020, those numbers had changed. Of the people surveyed, 11% still would not get vaccinated, and 24% were as yet undecided. (Perhaps the seriousness of the coronavirus had begun to be more widely recognized as time passed.) Some opposition to vaccines arose out of a mistrust of the government, a mistrust of science, and a mistrust of the pharmaceutical companies. The fear was that they might try to sell their vaccines (even if they were harmful) out of a desire to make a profit.

Now, a year and a half after the beginning of the pandemic, several COVID-19 vaccines have been produced, and the picture has changed somewhat. According to the Kaiser Family Foundation COVID Vaccine Monitor, an ongoing research project tracking the public's attitudes about the COVID-19 vaccine, a growing number of people are open to the idea of getting vaccinated. "The share of U.S. adults who want to get the vaccine has increased among Black, Hispanic, and White adults alike, and the share who say they want to 'wait and see' how it works for other people has declined among Black and White adults" (Hamel et al., 2021, p. 3).

Partisanship plays an important role in the public's attitudes toward COVID-19 vaccination. Democrats and independents have increased positive attitudes about vaccination, whereas Republicans remain the most resistant, with 33% stating they will not get the vaccine unless it is required for work, school, or other reasons (Hamel et al., 2021).

Unfortunately, racial and economic inequality figure prominently into the COVID-19 vaccine situation. According to Hamel et al. (2021), "Black and Hispanic adults and those with lower incomes are less likely than their White and higher-income counterparts to say they have personally received at least one dose of the vaccine or that they know someone who has" (p. 2). Knowing someone who has been vaccinated is correlated with both vaccine hesitance and enthusiasm. Among people who indicate they want the vaccine as soon as possible, about half know someone who has already been vaccinated. Among the people who indicate they will only get it if they are required to, only about 29% actually know someone who has already been vaccinated (Hamel et al., 2021).

The messaging related to the COVID-19 vaccines is extremely important, as it can have a big impact on the public's willingness to get vaccinated (or not). Messages that emphasize the effectiveness of the vaccines and their ability to prevent people from dying as well as the vaccines' role in helping society return to normal may motivate people to be immunized. Conversely, messages about allergic reactions and unpleasant side effects from the vaccines may be disincentives for people to become immunized (Hamel et al., 2021).

According to Redford (2021), in a discussion about myths and the COVID-19 vaccines, concerns were shared about the vaccines not covering the variants. Several variants have been shown to be "easily neutralized" by the current vaccines available. According to AAMC.org (2021), if one is vaccinated with any of the COVID-19 vaccines available now, there is protection against the 2020 strains and the Alpha variant. Other known variants such as the Beta variant and the Delta variant have not been as easily neutralized, but vaccines are not considered completely useless against them (para. 27). (The World Health Organization has relabeled COVID variants from numerical value to Greek names.)

Current Status of COVID-19 Vaccinations

As of August 2021, the fight against the spread of COVID-19 infection continues, and vaccine refusal has emerged as a huge public health issue. More than 93 million people are eligible but continue to refuse COVID-19 vaccines. There is no single answer to who is refusing the COVID-19 vaccines, but there appears to be two groups. One group is still deciding (waiting and watching). This group is made up mostly of African Americans, Latinx, and Democrats—usually urban and younger. Another group continues to vehemently refuse the vaccine. This second group tends to be white, rural, evangelical Christians who are politically conservative. Although these demographics might be changing, many organizations continue to study the composition of those who refuse vaccines in order to increase vaccination rates.

Overlapping fears include vaccine safety, conspiracy theories, disbelief in vaccine efficacy, and apprehension about side effects. Some believe they are invincible to the infection, describing their immune system as being strong and healthy enough to fight off the disease.

> Approximately 50% of the adult population in the United States has yet to receive a shot, and about 41.5% of youth ages 12–17 have yet to receive the shot (CDC, 2021a).
>
> As of July 30, 2021, due to fears about the rapidly spreading delta variant, injections were up from 500,000 to 652,000 doses on average each day. Although the trend of hospitalization did go down, this trend has resurfaced due to the delta variant. However, as of this writing, 97% of people hospitalized for COVID-19 were unvaccinated. Experts estimate that 90% or more of the adult and child population would need to be vaccinated to reach the herd immunity threshold (Gill, 2021).

DISTRUST OF VACCINES ON THE GLOBAL LEVEL

One systematic literature review of multiple databases from 2000 to February 2014 investigated vaccine hesitancy in low- and middle-income countries. After exclusion criteria were applied, there were 23 studies from countries in Asia, 16 studies from countries in Africa, four studies from South America, and one from Oceania (Munoz et al., 2015). The most frequently cited concern was the perception that vaccines could be harmful. The second-highest concern in the qualitative studies was that vaccines could be part of a global conspiracy against certain communities or religious groups (especially prevalent in some Muslim communities). Worries about the quality and cost of vaccines were frequently reported in the studies conducted across the African continent. Religious beliefs were also cited as being a source for lack of trust in vaccines (immunization being "against God's will"). Some studies cited people's unpleasant experiences with healthcare workers. Fears of receiving too many vaccines at once were also raised. It was felt that this could have a deleterious effect upon the immune system.

8 ADULT MEDICAL TREATMENT REFUSALS, LIMITATIONS, AND DELAYS

Although there is quite a lot of research about the reasons people refuse vaccination, little has been studied about effective interventions to address vaccine refusal. In these authors' experience, it is difficult to change the mind of a truly diehard anti-vaccinator, but those people who are "on the fence" may be willing to listen.

Suggestions for Communicating With Those Who Refuse Vaccines

- Ask them about their vaccine history.
- Try to address their hesitancy by finding out what keeps them from getting a recommended vaccine.
- Attempt to ease their fears and dispel any unfounded myths that they may raise.
- Use strong endorsements. Share that you have received that vaccination yourself and that you vaccinate your own family.
- Tell them that they cannot believe everything they read on the internet and that some of the information is false.
- Stress the risks and complications of the disease the vaccine is meant to prevent.
- Educate that vaccines not only prevent infections but also significant infection-related complications. For example, the flu vaccine lowers the risk of flu-related complications (e.g., hospitalizations, pneumonia).
- Remind patients that the flu vaccine may cause mild malaise or flu-like symptoms, but it does not cause the flu.
- Reassure them that studies consistently show that vaccines do not cause autism—not even the ones with thimerosal.

There are some structural measures one can take within primary care practices to increase immunization rates by holding primary care providers accountable during quarterly provider-level performance reports, implementing effective patient tracking and recall systems, providing provider education, analyzing missed opportunities, and devising ways to eliminate them (Loskutova et al., 2020). In addition, some primary care practices utilize incentives and rewards when care teams achieve the immunization benchmarks for their patient panels. Progress toward immunization and other benchmarks can be posted in the lunchroom or some other convenient place to foster an atmosphere of friendly competition among the care teams.

CHAPTER 9

OVERVIEW OF RELIGIOUS DOCTRINES

Several religious frameworks support refusal or limitation of medical care and treatments or prayer as the larger component of healing. In the data collected in this book, 42 separate churches that adhere to these limit or refusal frameworks were identified covering a historical time frame of 35 years. These religious frameworks were identified for their doctrines and teachings or their involvement with legal proceedings for child neglect. Not all religions have had children become gravely ill or die due to prayer in lieu of medical care, nor do all church members follow the doctrines or teachings of particular religions that promote withholding medical care for their members. The purpose of the latter part of this chapter is to present information from the literature, media, or interviews about religions that have been identified as having doctrines that influence healthcare decisions for children and/or adults. The intent is not to judge or make accusations. Rather, the intent is to inform healthcare professionals about identified religions or churches whose doctrines have potential to influence medical healthcare decisions.

Some churches embraced investigation; others would not return phone calls or letters of inquiry. Still others could not be located and were identified solely on the basis of legal or media summaries covering examples of treatment refusal and (sometimes) legal consequences.

CHURCHES WITH FRAMEWORKS SUPPORTING REFUSAL OF MEDICAL TREATMENT, LIMITATION, OR DELAY

The following list names 42 religious groups found in current literature whose doctrines or teachings have been noted to influence decisions about children's healthcare (Adams & Leverland, 1986; Asser & Swan, 1998; CHILD USA, n.d.; Massachusetts Citizens for Children, n.d.; Ontario Consultants on Religious Tolerance, n.d.; Swan, 1997, 2000, 2020a; Weller, 2017):

Jehovah's Witnesses

Christian Science

The Church of the Firstborn

Christian Catholic Church (not affiliated with the Roman Catholic Church)

Faith Assembly

Followers of Christ

Endtime Ministries

The Believers' Fellowship

Faith Temple Doctoral Church of Christ in God

The Source

Christ Miracle Healing Center

No Name Fellowship

The Fellowship

Faith Tabernacle Congregation

9 OVERVIEW OF RELIGIOUS DOCTRINES

Faith Temple Doctoral Church of Christ in God

1st Century Gospel Pentecostal Church

Evangelistic Healers

Jesus Through Jon and Judy

Wiccans (a group that identifies themselves as witches; not religious)

Four Square Church

Christ Assembly

The Church of God of the Union Assembly

Church of God Chapel

Northeast Kingdom Community Church

True Followers of Christ

Faith Cathedral Assembly

Faith Tabernacle

Living Word Assembly of God

Traveling Ministries Everyday Church

Bible Reading Fellowship

The Body (aka The Body of Christ)

Church of God Chapel

Amish

Scientologists

Mennonites

Unleavened Bread Ministries (online church)

Full Gospel Deliverance Church

Born in Zion Ministry

One Mind Ministries

Twelve Tribes

The Believers' Fellowship

Kostinchuk (2001) offers brief examples of a number of the religions on this list. In his descriptions of their beliefs, he sheds light on how these religions receive public awareness. He titles them the "players" and offers this information with numerous helpful references:

1. The Bible Reading Fellowship evangelical group located in California does not report or record births or deaths as required by state law. The group supports avoidance of all medical treatments.

2. Members of the sect Endtime Ministries hold faith healing as a high belief. They reject medical interventions for their children and do not allow healthcare professionals to be present at the birth of their babies.

3. Members of the Oregon-based Christ Church believe in the power of prayer as a cure for medical conditions. They prefer to use anointing oils and "laying on of hands" rather than traditional medical interventions, even for their children.

4. Many Pentecostal sects also believe in the "laying on of hands" rather than seeking medical attention for their members (including children).

5. Faith Tabernacle Congregation Church members believe that members can be cured of sickness by the prayers of "true believers." Members who seek medical care are seen by some members as turning their backs on God and their faith.

6. According to followers of the General Assembly Church of the Firstborn, the sovereign power of God to heal is the center of their belief system.

7. Members of the Faith Tabernacle Congregation Church are encouraged to follow what the group sees as God's will, including the notion that God's will is not to seek medical treatment, even for church members' children.

Unfortunately, most of the 42 religious groups listed on the previous pages do not have accessible information about the particulars of their religious doctrines. When a healthcare professional encounters a "family of faith" about whom there is little knowledge, the best source of information will be the family itself. With great respect toward privacy, the professional healthcare provider should ask probing questions to assess the family's individualized interpretation of the belief system, using a tone of acceptance. If fear arises, the opportunity for subsequent conversations or precious negotiations may be lost. Keep in mind that many people within religions believe in prayer and supernatural healing as a possibility. For the majority of people, medical care is readily accepted along with spiritual practices.

TYPES OF PRAYER AND RELIGIOSITY THAT INFLUENCE CHILDREN'S HEALTHCARE DECISIONS

As the use of integrated holistic and alternative health treatment continues to grow, there has been a great deal of attention given to the influence of religion, prayer, and consciousness on treatment decisions and health outcomes.

The study of the influence of religiosity on healthcare decisions dates back to the 19th century (1872) and was addressed in a systematic review of original research by Koenig (2012). He identified 454 studies. Few of the studies published were explicitly designed to investigate religion. Rather, most were intended to identify the relationship of health outcomes, morbidity, and mortality to one or more religious indicators.

According to Levin (1994), medicine has not historically recognized that one's religious background is influential to one's healthcare decisions. "As a result, the idea that one's religious background or experiences might in some way influence one's health has remained part of the folklore of discussion on the fringes of the research community" (p. 1475).

The Institute of Noetic Studies, located in Northern California, conducted empirical research on the power of prayer (also called *intention* by Noetic members) in healing, including experiments on the results of local and distant prayer (intention) on physiological measurements (Issues on Spirituality and Research Lecture Series,

2001, personal communication, Gayle Swift, Dominican University of California).

Dr. Jeffery S. Levin, a former medical school professor and epidemiologist, has published several articles seeking to validate the relationship between prayer and health. His articles review evidence found within hundreds of epidemiologic studies that have reported statistically significant findings (which he calls *salutary effects*) between religious indicators on reported morbidity and mortality. His research has led to the development of further questions including "Is it valid?" and "Is it causal?" His research has led to evidence that says "yes," "probably," and "maybe" (Levin, 1994). Levin continued to study the connection between faith and healing and has published five books, several based on international research, in the areas of the relationship among faith, healing, and prayer. According to Levin (1994), questions still posed include:

1. What is the transcendence experience?
2. What is the role of faith, spirituality, and healing?
3. Can the transcendence experience be studied?
4. How can religious faith serve as a resource for the prevention of illness and the promotion of well-being?

A final causal summation remains difficult.

Levin's (1994) extensive review of hundreds of published research articles on the relationship between religiosity and health identified many confounding variables, including:

1. Strict lifestyle or health-related behaviors sanctioned by religious denominations.
2. Heredity as morbidity and mortality may be higher (or lower) in particular groups of people with shared religious beliefs (Tay-Sachs disease in Ashkenazi Jews, sickle cell anemia in

9 OVERVIEW OF RELIGIOUS DOCTRINES

Blacks, and hypercholesterolemia in Dutch Reformed Afrikaners).

3. Psychosocial effects, since many religious denominations provide intense social support, possibly buffering anger and stress.
4. Psychodynamics of belief systems that may engender purpose, peacefulness, and self-confidence (or the alternative).

Psychodynamics of faith, or the mere belief that religious beliefs of God are health-enhancing, may be enough to produce salutary effects (Levin, 1994).

One example shared in Levin's article (1994) is the lower incidence of hypertension found in several religious groups. One church noted to have healthier members than other religious groups are the Seventh-Day Adventists. A shared doctrine of not eating meat may contribute to a reduction of hypertension. Additionally, other doctrines of religious fellowship, self-responsibility, family solidarity, and self-care may contribute to beneficial health-related behaviors. Literature suggests that there may be a religion-health connection. For example, in a well-known study conducted from 2001 to 2007, known as the Adventist Health Study (AHS-2), with 96,000 subjects ranging from 30 to 112 years of age from all 50 states, data showed that those who participated in vegan diets had significantly lower BMIs than non-vegans and showed trends of lower cholesterol levels, lower rates of high blood pressure, and lower rates of diabetes (Loma Linda University Health, n.d.-a).

In general, the study of prayer as a healing tool poses problems and challenges for both the court systems, which have the responsibility to distinguish the validity of prayer as an alternative for medical care, and for researchers, who are seeking to validate prayer through such means as clinical trials. According to Dusek et al. (2003), there is an absence of knowledge and tangible evidence, or even the mechanism of a healing energy (or force) with prayer. These authors describe how the conduction of prospective randomized controlled clinical trials may truly not be necessary if the primary objective of a research study is to discover the philosophical underpinnings. According to the authors, the application of clinical trial designs poses the risk of being "overly reductionistic and detrimental." They offer two central assumptions (Dusek et al., 2003):

- Therapy studies should be definable enough to be integrated into a variety of healthcare systems.
- Research findings on the therapeutic impact on the combined mind-body-spirit continuum should include some measurable somatic component.

The research on prayer efficacy remains wide open. Some researchers have used high quality methods and others have not. Some of the reports using high quality clinical trials have demonstrated positive treatment effects, while others show no effect of prayer on healing. No clear patterns have emerged demonstrating which clinical conditions are most responsive to the effects of prayer, as most research has been conducted with "considerable heterogeneity of diseases that have been studied" (Dusek et al., 2003, p. A45).

One needs to ask whether prayer can indeed be scientifically studied as an actual healthcare intervention. With this question in mind, three distinct problems (among others) have emerged in the study of prayer (Dusek et al., 2003):

1. The theological concerns that prayer studies attempt to manipulate God or reduce divine influence to equations seeking causal relationships
2. The scientific concerns over the absence of plausible or known mechanisms for which healing prayer might actually influence health
3. The concerns over the definition of "dose of prayer" and the concerns over the manner in which the prayer is provided

There have been no concrete suggestions put forth in current research literature to guide researchers through these problems. Research continues to be conducted with a milieu of interventional mechanisms.

CLERICAL INTERPRETATIONS

Prayer itself has been defined in many ways. The following sections are devoted to definitions of various types of prayer, including clerical definitions, how the prayer is constructed, and how the prayer might be offered.

PRAYER AS AN ALTERNATIVE OR COMPLEMENTARY THERAPY

Prayer has been considered as an alternative or an adjunct to allopathic Western medical care for decades. Only recently has prayer become a center of empirical study. People of diverse cultures and associations have used prayer as an alternative or in conjunction with treatments with tremendously successful testimonies. Prayer can be distant or it can be bedside. It can be individualized or it can be applied in groups.

According to Dr. Michael Lerner, who served as President of Commonweal and co-creator of the Commonweal Cancer Help Program in Bolinas, California, prayer has been studied as an adjunct to allopathic Western medical care to identify its therapeutic effects. In *Choices in Healing: Integrating the Best of Conventional and Complementary Approaches to Cancer* (1994), Lerner describes the outcome of a study performed by Dr. Randolph Byrd, carried out at the San Francisco General Medical Center. Byrd's research was to determine whether antirecessionary prayer (prayer for a patient by others) offered by born-again Christians, as described by the Gospel of John 3:3, offered a therapeutic effect in conjunction with traditional prayer.

The study found that six conditions improved. The conditions were:

1. The need for intubation or ventilation
2. The need for antibiotics
3. The incidence of cardiopulmonary arrest
4. The incidence of congestive heart failure
5. The incidence of pneumonia
6. The need for diuretics

The study group ($N = 393$, 192 in the intervention group and 201 in the control group) demonstrated a general tendency for better physical outcomes than those who were not prayed for (Lerner, 1994).

FAITH HEALING

Religious affiliations promoting faith-healing measures to the exclusion of medical care are not new. Faith healing has been well documented in the literature for over 200 years. An example of faith-healing sects is the General Assembly Church of the Firstborn, whose members consider it a sin to seek medical care above God's power to heal. Amanda Bates, whose parents were part of the General Assembly Church of the Firstborn in Colorado, died of complications of untreated diabetes while her parents prayed over her (Dyer, 2000). Another example of an application of faith-healing concerns a religious group-healing procedure given to an adolescent who complained of a migraine headache:

> The group of faithful adults circled the child and described to her that her headaches were not real; rather, they were the results of sinful behaviors and sinful thoughts. The leader of the group continued to 'praise God for His amazing power of healing' and 'shunned the devil from causing pain and disease in the natural world.' The child was

instructed to ask for forgiveness, keeping her eyes closed while the group 'laid on' healing hands. At the conclusion of the prayer session, the girl remained calm, eyes closed for a long period of time, and reported that the headache was resolving. They kept her in bed for an hour or more after the healing session. (H. Conrad, personal communication, May 24th, 2005)

Faith healings can take place in dyads, small groups, or large staged gatherings. Sometimes cults or religious groups will charge an entry fee for attending faith-healing sessions. The one being healed may pay more for the cure.

Prayer is a complex human interest that can be viewed through many different lenses. Prayer used for healing has a special lens, since those who participate have a particular goal—to call upon external forces to provide care, healing, support, comfort, direction, and evidence of presence and relationship.

SPECIFIC RELIGIOUS DOCTRINES DEFINED

Of the 42 previously listed religions with doctrines that reference parents' healthcare decisions for their children, not all can be substantiated or validated through reputable sources. Therefore, the following sections include descriptions only for the most prevalent doctrines that are verifiable via reputable sources in the literature.

It is important to reinforce that not all church members follow such influential church doctrines. Nor do all of the individual churches listed earlier in this chapter teach the doctrines, faith-healing practices, or prayer sessions that may influence healthcare decisions that could ultimately endanger children's and adults' lives. Individual congregational members may adopt behaviors, beliefs, and values based on their own interpretation of biblical passages, or they may follow the lead of strict or radical church members or leaders who are highly influential regarding the adherence of religious teachings and healthcare decisions.

The first two church doctrines we describe are from the Jehovah's Witness church and the Christian Science church. These churches are reputable institutions with a worldwide membership base, both of which have doctrines that highly influence treatment decisions. Following these presentations, we briefly describe an evangelical church. The selection of the churches we discuss was based solely on the amount of legitimate and reputable sources of literature found.

JEHOVAH'S WITNESSES

In 1872, the Jehovah's Witness (JW) sect was built as a nondenominational study group by Charles Taze Russell (1852–1916), a Pennsylvanian, during the Adventist movement. By 1909, this first study group spawned study groups all over the world that focused on biblical prophecy, and thus the Watchtower Bible and Tract Society—the official name of the JW organization—was international. Currently, there are 2.5 million followers as of 2015 statistics in the US (Melton, 2014). JWs have distinguished themselves by being nontrinitarian and creating their own doctrine, called New World Translation of the Holy Spirit, which is based on interpretations of the Bible. In 1927, the first biblical publication was disseminated forbidding blood transfusion on penalty of loss of eternal life in God's kingdom (Vercillo & Duprey, 1988); by 1931, the organization officially acquired the name (Chand et al., 2014); and in 1945, the governing organization of JW first introduced the restriction on blood transfusions (Chand et al., 2014). According to Panico, Jenq, and Brewster (2011) and Melton (2014), JW is one of the fastest growing religions in the US. International membership in JW continues to grow rapidly. JW has

9 OVERVIEW OF RELIGIOUS DOCTRINES

interpreted the most frequently cited verses of the Bible as making references that (Thurkauf, 1989):

> "Every moving thing that lives shall be food for you . . . only you shall not eat flesh with its life, that is, its blood" (Genesis 8: 3–4).

> "For it has seemed good to the Holy Spirit and to us to lay upon you . . . these necessary things: that you abstain from what has been sacrificed to idols and from blood" (Acts 15: 28–29).

> "You must not eat the blood of any sort of flesh, because the soul of every sort of flesh is its blood. Anyone eating it will be cut off" (Leviticus 17: 13–14).

Denouncement of blood transfusions by the Watchtower Society took place in the 1940s. According to Swan (1997), the timing was curious in that during that time period, JWs were refusing to sing the national anthem. Swan (1997) describes that in the 1940s, media coverage emphasized that donating blood was a patriotic duty.

The underlying theme to JW teachings is the consequences of disobedience. According to Quintero (1993, p. 46), their belief system states:

> that if God's directive is not obeyed, eternal life is forfeited. If they disobey God and are 'cut-off,' believers will be denied life through resurrection. If a person's life is extended by a transfusion, it will become meaningless and lack spiritual purpose because the hope of everlasting life has been forfeited.

The idea that the soul of one is its blood was first given to Noah. Witnesses believe they apply to all humankind because all humankind is Noah's family (Thurkauf, 1989).

As described by Quintero's (1993) article on blood administration in pediatrics, JWs believe that violation means loss of salvation, and some insist that the negative spiritual effects are incurred regardless of whether the person actually chooses the blood transfusion. Other JWs disagree and assert that if you are unconscious, or it is transfused against one's will, the soul is not affected. In certain cases, members are shunned from their religious community and taught to believe they will no longer be able to enter eternal life (Panico et al., 2011).

In the article titled "Refusal of Medical Blood Transfusion Among Jehovah's Witnesses: Emotion Regulation of the Dissonance of Saving and Sacrificing Life," Ringnes and Hegstad (2016) discuss the implications of religion and the psychosocial effects it has on health decisions, and they analyze what it means to refuse blood products when death is preventable. JW's refusal of transfusion is the ultimate act of devotion to the church. In the perception of family and loved ones it can be an act of heroism and commitment to the faith. The article explains a thematic analysis that was conducted in 2011. Data were collected from multiple sources, specifically interviews, participants, observation, and texts. Results concluded that the study could not identify any clear conclusions if the emotion regulation strategies resolve the cognitive dissonance at the individual level (Ringnes & Hegstad, 2016). Researchers identified a life-death cognitive dissonance presented in the article as the focus on eternal life versus the possibility of accepting a blood transfusion and not dying now but giving up the chance for eternal life.

The challenge for healthcare professionals is not that JWs believe genuinely that they have responsibility for their child's food, shelter, and healthcare (Quintero, 1993), but that their faith will allow their own child's death before they would go against their interpretation of the Bible and consent for transfusion (Vercillo & Dupery, 1988). They will defend their right to make medical decisions for their children on the basis that, as parents, they are responsible adults (Quintero, 1993).

With all the pharmaceutical and technological progress we encounter daily in the healthcare arena, there are still very few alternatives to blood transfusion. (See Table 9.1 for a summary of the latest approaches and techniques in this area.) Based on literature reports, conflicts exist within the JW community, as some adherents will accept blood-based treatments but not blood itself (Muramoto, 1999). See Table 9.2 for a list of components and procedures acceptable or unacceptable within the JW faith, compiled from Watchtower Society publications and from statements by JW physicians.

Here lies the conflict: How should the healthcare professional proceed? Should one respect the deeply held beliefs of the parents or save the child's life? Modern technology is moving to help the health sciences and loving families, as there are now a number of alternatives to blood transfusions.

Table 9.1 Blood Transfusion Alternatives

Alternative Approach	Techniques
Maximize blood production	Erythropoietin
	Intravenous iron dextran
	Nutritional support including calories and amino acids for red blood cell production
Maximize cardiac output	Volume expansion via synthetic colloids and crystalloid solutions such as:
	Hydroxyethyl starch
	Dextran 40 and Dextran 70
	Urea-bridged gelatin
	Modified fluid gelatin
	Hemodilution

continues

Table 9.1 Blood Transfusion Alternatives (cont.)

Alternative Approach	Techniques
Increase oxygen content	Oxygen
	Fluorinated blood substitutes that carry oxygen
	Red blood cell substitutes:
	Perfluorocarbons
	Hb solutions such as Hb-based oxygen carriers, which are "chemically modified Hb solutions containing polymerized, conjugated, or liposome-encapsulated Hb" (not yet FDA approved; Chand et al., 2014, p. 661)
Decrease metabolic rate	Hypothermia (targeting core temperatures of 30–32° C to reduce oxygen consumption by 40%)
	Paralysis with ventilator support to prevent oxygen consuming shivering
Minimize blood losses	Microchemistry analyzers
	Pediatric-sized blood samples
	Sterile reservoirs
	Hypotensive anesthesia in intra-operative procedures
	Desmopressin to reduce blood loss after cardiopulmonary bypass surgery

Surgical procedures	Local infiltration with vasopressors
	Preliminary ligation of major arteries
Hypotensive anesthesia	Deliberate reduction of systolic blood pressure to 80–90 mmHg, decreased mean arterial pressure (MAP) to 50–65 mmHg (or the reduction of MAP by 30% of patient's baseline) via pharmacologic agents such as sevoflurane, isoflurane, halothane, vasodilators such as nitroglycerine and adenosine, and/or clonidine, calcium channel blockers, angiotensin converting enzyme inhibitors, and others
Continuing or yet to be developed	Genetically engineered pig hemoglobin solutions
	Human hemoglobin solutions
	Longer half-life solutions of fluorocarbon preparations

Table 9.2 Blood Product–Related Procedures Acceptable or Unacceptable to Jehovah's Witnesses

Blood Product	Stance in Accordance with Jehovah's Witness Beliefs
Whole blood	Unacceptable if taken as "blood transfusion"
	Acceptable if taken as contained in bone marrow transplant
	Many refuse preoperative autologous donation

continues

Table 9.2 Blood Product–Related Procedures Acceptable or Unacceptable to Jehovah's Witnesses (cont.)

Blood Product	Stance in Accordance with Jehovah's Witness Beliefs
Plasma proteins	Unacceptable if taken as "plasma"
	Acceptable if taken separately as individual blood components such as albumin, clotting factors, or fibrin
	Unacceptable if considered unfractionated plasma
	Acceptable if taken as albumin or albumin solutions
	Acceptable if taken as cryoprecipitate, clotting factor concentrates, fibrinogen concentrates, and immunoglobins
White blood cell transfusion	Unacceptable if taken as "white blood cell transfusion"
	Acceptable if taken as "peripheral stem cell transfusion"
Autologous blood	Unacceptable if tube connection to the patient's body is interrupted
	Acceptable if the tube to the body is maintained such as hemodilution or a cell-saver machine to capture and re-infuse one's blood during or after surgical procedures
Stem cell transfusion	Unacceptable if taken from the umbilical cord blood
	Acceptable if taken from peripheral circulation or bone marrow

Heart-lung machine technology	Unacceptable if patient's blood is used to prime the machine
	Acceptable if the patient's blood is used to circulate the machine after priming
Epidural blood patch	Unacceptable if blood is removed from the vein and injected back into the patient
	Acceptable if the blood is injected through a syringe that is connected to the vein via a continuous tube system
Blood donations	Unacceptable if the blood is donated by Jehovah's Witnesses for use by other Jehovah's Witnesses and others
	Acceptable if donated by non-JWs for use by JWs and others (and only for use of blood components, not as packed cell transfusion, whole blood transfusion, or other intact blood in its non-single component form)
Other	Usually there is no objection to intraoperative cell salvage, hemodialysis, apheresis, cardiac bypass procedures
	Usually there is no objection to iron, tranexamic acid, and agents that stimulate erythropoiesis or granulocyte colony stimulating factors
	Generally acceptable: recombinant factor VIIa
	"Matters of conscience" (Chand, Subramanya, & Rao, 2014): platelets, clotting factors, albumin, cell savers, epidural blood patches, and immunoglobulins

(Joint United Kingdom Blood Transfusion and Tissue Transplantation Services Professional Advisory Committee [JPAC], 2020b; Muramoto, 1999, p. 298)

Status of Acceptability of Procedures for Jehovah's Witnesses

According to the latest literature, there is a range of acceptability of transfusion products and procedures. The following list describes which procedures and products are generally accepted, generally not accepted, and those left up to individual decisions:

Generally accepted:

- Crystalloid intravenous solutions (for blood volume expansion): ringer's lactate, normal saline solutions, hypertonic saline solutions
- Colloids (used to replace lost plasma proteins): dextran, gelatin, hetastarch
- Perfluorochemicals (chemicals used in the lungs to increase oxygen/carbon dioxide exchange)
- Erythropoietin (medication used to promote the production of red blood cells from the bone marrow)
- Thrombopoietin mimetics (increases the production of platelets by stimulating the cell receptor for thrombopoietin, a natural hormone)
- Administration of tranexamic acid (antifibrinolytic) which can reduce mortality during hemorrhages related to trauma, gastric hemorrhages, and obstetric hemorrhages

Generally not accepted:

- Whole blood transfusions (may be used during emergencies to quickly restore blood volume)

- Packed red blood cell transfusions (most frequently used form of transfusion therapy)
- Leukocyte transfusions (used in extreme states of neutropenia to boost the immune system)
- Plasma (used for clotting factors and infrequently used for blood volume expansion)
- Auto-transfusions (used when one's condition allows the collection and banking of one's own blood for later use, thus reducing the chances of being exposed to the foreign proteins or possible infectious diseases that one can be exposed to during donated blood transfusions)
- Preoperative cell salvage and reinfusion
- Postoperative cell salvage and reinfusion

Left up to individual decision:

- Cardiopulmonary bypass technology (used for cardiac and pulmonary emergencies and surgeries)

(JPAC, 2020a; Mann et al., 1992, p. 1043)

The conflict surrounding freedom of choice for JWs has been presented in literature by Muramoto (1999). He reports that the Watch Tower Society does not give church members the freedom to accept blood therapy without penalty. According to Muramoto, a JW who accepts a blood-based product and does not repent of the action before a judicial committee will receive the harshest sanction of the religion: disfellowship or excommunication. Because accepting transfusions is considered betraying God, the offender will be socially isolated and shunned by church members.

In contrast, Heller (2005) reports that the JW church members do not censure members who choose to take another course (seeking transfusions). He quotes James Pellechia, director of public affairs for JW, as saying: "We believe in seeking the best medical help for ourselves and our families. It is the Christian thing to do. If someone caves under pressure, we offer aid and support, do what we can pastorally to help the family" (p. 2).

When dealing with blood transfusions situations involving JWs, it is critical for the healthcare team to demonstrate that the blood transfusion (or blood product) is lifesaving. Courts have been known to refuse a petition for an order for JW children with sickle cell disease and JW children who need preoperative or intra-operative transfusion (Quintero, 1993). According to Winiarski, Klatt, and Kazerouninia (2018), courts, when confronted by families refusing lifesaving transfusions for a child, continue to uphold the hospital's ability to provide blood against a Jehovah's Witness's parent's desires. These authors state that when a court order is sought, it only relates to the transfusion of the blood product while the parents retain all other parental rights. "When court is involved, a parent sometimes mistakenly believes that their parental rights are broadly being taken away, a distressing misconception" (para. 16).

Many JWs seek "contracts" from their physicians that no blood products will be transfused under any conditions. Alternatively, church members have been known to sign a statement agreeing to absolve the physician and healthcare team from all responsibility. When it comes to children's immediate healthcare needs during times of life-or-death decision-making, physicians may not accept these statements and instead may continue to petition to the courts for temporary legal guardianship so that transfusion therapy can ensue. According to Migden and Braen (1998), it is general practice that adult JWs carry with them a card that speaks to their desire to refuse blood, even if deemed lifesaving by the attending physician.

9 OVERVIEW OF RELIGIOUS DOCTRINES

In 1998, there were over 3.2 million JWs worldwide, of which 25% resided in the US. In 2002, there were more than 6 million worldwide, with 1 million in the US and 100,000 in Canada, including hundreds of healthcare professionals, surgeons, and physicians. In 2020, there were reported to be 8,695,808 adherents worldwide (JW.org, 2021).

What these statistics reinforce is that healthcare professionals must be fully aware of the need to meticulously assess the situations and deem the treatment lifesaving before petitioning to the courts. All alternatives to blood transfusion and all alternatives to those treatments considered unacceptable to the church must be considered prior to transfusion. Whenever possible, in emergency and non-emergency situations, clergy and family members should be consulted prior to proceeding with standard transfusion therapy.

There is now a growing group within the greater JW membership that is pushing to reform the church's stance on transfusion therapy. The group, known as Associated Jehovah's Witnesses for Reform on Blood (or AJWRB), has a website (www.ajwrb.org) that discusses reform issues. As quoted from the site: "In former times thousands of youths died for putting God first. They are still doing it, only today the drama is played out in hospitals and courtrooms, with blood transfusions the issue" (AJWRB, 1994, p. 2). The website continues with a description that some JWs believe that "a blood transfusion is a liquid tissue or organ transplant, not a meal, and hence does not violate the biblical admonition to abstain from (eating) blood" (AJWRB, 2017).

AJWRB, an international group representing members in many countries, calls for its members and other leaders to be child advocates. The group encourages questioning those JW members who go door to door to explain how the Watchtower (the leadership base of JW) decides "which parts of blood God permits" (AJWRB, n.d.). The AJWRB calls for a termination of subsidizing the Watchtower Society's continued desire for legal exemptions, and the site requires that children's medical needs continue to be protected. The site also has a brief critique of a previously published *AWAKE!* magazine (published by the Watchtower Society, May 22, 1994) that featured 26 children who did not receive blood transfusions due to religious exemption and did not survive. The President of the Constitutional Court of Colombia, Dr. Vladimiro Naranjo, states: "This is a form of murder, moreover, First Degree Murder" (AJWRB.org, 1998, para. 10). In other words, he considers the loss of children's lives directly related to blood transfusion refusal to be first-degree murder.

JW has a strong international presence and seems to place significant value on the discussion of its beliefs, as witnessed firsthand by those who have been visited by JWs. According to Thurkauf (1989), JWs will be grateful if their beliefs are honored. The stress and anxiety of serious illness are still realities, and it is very important to continue to provide support in a nonjudgmental way. Tables 9.1 and 9.2 earlier in the chapter provide a thorough overview of allowed and disallowed blood-based treatments. Knowledge of these policies can be very helpful to healthcare professionals faced with a blood transfusion refusal, as it will help the family feel more understood and less judged. Thus, this knowledge will help keep stress as low as possible during discussion and negotiations for necessary treatments. It is important to remember that for the family, making these decisions isn't easy, and supportive environments can go a long way toward easing the situation.

CHRISTIAN SCIENTISTS

Mary Baker Eddy established the religious doctrine of the Church of Christ, Scientist—typically known as Christian Science—in 1879. Church doctrines were based upon her own "divine" healing, which occurred in 1866 after reading the New Testament's disclosure of Jesus's healing practices (christianscience.com, 2021a). In 1875, she wrote a book, *Science and Health,* which was later published as *Science and Health, With Key to the Scripture.* This text describes the principles of divine healing and laws expressed in the acts and sayings of Jesus. Christian Science teaches that God is the only reality and that one can overcome sin, evil, and illness by understanding this principle. The teachings of Eddy clearly describe reliance on spiritual rather than medical means for healing. Each church is self-governed and without individual pastors; two readers conduct each service with universally shared lessons, culled mainly from Eddy's book.

Numerous publications are the guiding communication of Christian Science beliefs. These publications include *The Christian Science Monitor*, *Christian Science Quarterly* Bible Lessons, the *Christian Science Sentinel*, *The Herald of Christian Science*, and *The Christian Science Journal* (The First Church of Christ, Scientist, n.d.). See the nearby sidebar with quotes from Eddy's 1875 book and 1925 teachings, which succinctly describe her doctrine.

Mary Baker Eddy Quotes

The prayer of faith shall save the sick, says the scripture. What is this healing prayer? A mere request that God will heal the sick has no power to gain more of the divine presence than is always at hand. The beneficial effect of such prayer for the sick is on the human mind, making it act more powerfully on the body through a blind faith in God. (Eddy, 1875, p. 12)

The proof of Truth, life and love, which Jesus gave by casting out error and healing the sick, completed his earthly mission; but in the Christian Church this demonstration of healing was early lost, about three centuries after the crucifixion. No ancient school of philosophy, material medica, or scholastic theology ever taught or demonstrated the divine healing of absolute science. (Eddy, 1875, p. 41)

After a lengthy examination of my discovery and its demonstration in healing the sick, this fact became evident to me—that the mind governs the body, not partially but wholly. I submitted my metaphysical system of treating disease to the broadest practical tests. Since then this system has gradually gained ground, and has proved itself,

> whenever scientifically employed, to be the most effective curative agent in medical practice. (Eddy, 1875, p. 112)
>
> Disease being a belief, a latent illusion of mortal mind, the sensation would not appear if the error of belief was met and destroyed by truth. If we understand the control of mind over body, we should put no faith in material means . . . drugs and medicine. (Eddy, 1875, pp. 168–169)
>
> A patient hears the doctor's verdict as a criminal hears his death sentence. The patient may seem calm under it, but he is not. His fortitude may sustain him, not his fear, which has already developed the disease that is gaining the mastery, is increased by the physician's words. (Eddy, 1875, p. 198)

A complex component of Christian Science is the church's communications to its practitioners and "nurses." According to Christianscience.com (2021b), Christian Science nursing is considered skillful, practical healing assistance and care to one in need. A nurse is a member of the "Mother Church" who understands and implements wisdom in a sick room. Care is consistent with theology and is limited to bathing, mobility, nourishment, and cleansing bandages but does not include medications or any medically oriented technology, as nurses are to avoid administering any type of medicine or conducting behaviors that could be interpreted as practicing medicine (Christianscience.com, 2021b).

According to Swan (1997), the religion also has tenets that discourage reporting of sick children who have had medical treatment refused or withheld, even though Christian Science practitioners are not exempt from state-mandated child abuse reporting for the withholding of medical treatment. Reporting suspected communicable diseases to health officials has also been discouraged. This puts healthcare professionals at a disadvantage in treating children who have been identified

9 OVERVIEW OF RELIGIOUS DOCTRINES

as needing healthcare, yet it allows the church members a chance to apply their scientific prayer in lieu of traditional medical care.

What happens when the prayer administered by faithful Christian Scientists does not work to cure disease? Swan (1997) reports that the Christian Science "nurses" have attended children who have died of meningitis, pneumonia, diabetes, and bowel obstructions. Reimbursement by third-party payers has been established in some states. A Blue Cross representative noted that, like psychiatric care, treatments by Christian Science practitioners is justified. Furthermore, Medicare, Medicaid, and many plans for government employees have historically covered practitioner treatments (Swan, 1997). According to Christianscience.com (2020, para. 1–2):

> Various U.S. federal, state, and private health insurance plans provide for the reimbursement of Christian Science nursing care and practitioner treatment. The U.S. Federal Office has been working to increase the availability of insurance options that cover these types of care. Thirteen Christian Science nursing facilities across the United States are Medicare providers.

Of interest are the state laws that exist that allow exemptions of Christian Science children in studying about diseases. The church claims that teaching children about disease and disease-related symptoms tends to undermine the teachings of the doctrine (Swan, 1997). Although the American Medical Association (2019) has called for a removal of statutes giving religious exemptions from immunizations, no legislation has been passed to repeal them. All 50 states now have legislation requiring specified vaccines for students; however, they also have exemptions for students who have medical reasons. There are 45 states, and Washington, DC, that continue to grant religious exemptions for those with religious objections, and 15 states that allow for philosophical exemptions such as moral or personal beliefs (Immunization Action Coalition, 2019; NCSL.org, 2020).

The Christian Science church circulates lists of diseases that are required to be reported to health authorities and encourages their family members to follow the law and report them. In contradiction, the church does not describe the reportable diseases and claims that "ignorance of disease is desirable in healing it spiritually and warns against getting a medical diagnosis" (Swan, 1997, p. 500).

A position paper was published in *The New England Journal of Medicine* in 1983 by the Christian Science church. Several of the sentiments that relate to the church's beliefs and doctrines concerning children and healthcare are shared in the nearby sidebar.

Christian Science Church Beliefs and Doctrines

According to an article by Nathan Talbot (1983) in *The New England Journal of Medicine:*

> Christian Scientists are caring and responsible people who love their children and want only the best possible care for them. They would not have relied on Christian Science for healing—sometimes over four and even five generations in the same family—if this healing were only a myth. Yet they approach the subject of healing on the basis of a very different perspective from that of medical practice. (p. 1641)

> To them it is part of a whole religious way of life and is, in fact, the natural outcome of theology that underlies it. This theology, Christian Scientists believe, is both biblically based and deeply reasoned. Indeed, they speak of it as "scientific" because they believe its truth has been demonstrated through practical healing experience time and time again. Certainly, Christian Science is leagues apart from faith-healing groups that have aroused current concerns, and its adherents share neither the fundamentalist theology nor the rigidly proscriptive views of

medicine characteristic of these groups. They are given neither to blind invoking of "miracles" nor passive submission to sickness as God's will. (p. 1641)

If a patient decides to turn to medical care, the Christian Science practitioner—in the patient's own interests—releases the case in a supportive spirit and without reproach. And if a Christian Scientist decides on medical treatment, he or she should cooperate with the physician without entertaining mental reservations about the treatment, which, as many doctors might acknowledge, could be detrimental to its effectiveness. (p. 1643)

Furthermore, members of this denomination take community concerns about the well-being of children with deep seriousness. They have a strong record of cooperation with public-health officials over the years . . . Christian Science parents would not object to the administration of on-the-spot first aid for their children. But in some instances they might prefer, after careful consideration, to have Christian Science treatment rather than hospitalization, surgery, or extended therapy. Again, however, prayer and reasoned judgment amid the exigencies of practical situations—rather than abstract criteria—tend to shape the choice of treatment in emergency situations . . . Christian Scientists also obey the law when vaccination is required (though requesting exemption when it is possible), and they have a physician or licensed midwife in attendance at childbirth. (p. 1643)

The only purpose of Christian Scientists' work with legislators has been to ensure that the responsible use of prayer on behalf of children is not equated with abuse and neglect. Our society should consider very carefully just how far it is prepared to go in the direction of claiming to determine that the emphasis on spiritual healing in the New Testament must be held so suspect that it should be

> virtually proscribed by law. Christian Scientists believe that within the framework of existing law, states can adequately protect children without arbitrarily intruding on parental rights or abridging religious rights that are important to all. (p. 1644)

There is no doubt that Christian Science parents love and care for their children. The adherence to the faithful perspective that disease does not exist, should not be named, and should not be treated with traditional medical care before prayer does influence the relationship among healthcare providers, public health officials, teachers, and families. The view that this is neglect or abuse must be looked at critically for each case encountered, and families should be supported in their care and concern for their children's welfare as well as their relationship with God. Healthcare professionals must balance parents' desires to pray for their child, bring in a Christian Science practitioner, and have the time to offer their services prior to instigating traditional treatment, but not at the expense of the child's wellness or life. Legislative battles continue concerning upholding medical exemptions for families of faith or concerning the proposed adoption of new exemption legislation; therefore, healthcare professionals of all disciplines must be aware of the religious tenets of this faith and be prepared to act immediately on behalf of the child.

FOLLOWERS OF CHRIST CHURCH

The Followers of Christ Church are a faithful group with wide representation. In his article "The Battle Over Faith Healing," Mark Larabee, a reporter for *The Oregonian* (1998), reports how the Followers of Christ Church in Oregon City amassed one of the largest faith-healing child death concentrations identified in the US. A Followers of Christ Church member interviewed by Larabee describes a Christ- and Bible-stressing, tight-knit sect of Christian Bible believers who encourage strict loyalty, an ardent faith in God and in divine

9 OVERVIEW OF RELIGIOUS DOCTRINES

healing, acceptance of the Lord's chastening as a parent's loving spanking, and suspicion of worldly outsiders. Members rely on the prayer closet (meetings of faithful members to apply faith-healing services directed by the pastor) and on faith healing as Christ's channel of deliverance from evils of all kinds.

Web-based reports can be found that describe the significant details of the child losses of members of the Followers of Christ Church. The Culteducationinstitute.com (2014) website has a comprehensive listing of cases that the Cult Education Institute gathered about the Followers of Christ and other faith-healing churches. The Followers of Christ Church was established in Oregon and has a presence in other western states, including a large population in Idaho. One prominent belief is that members are to rely on God's healing rather than on modern medicine and physicians. This type of healing is for sickness and injury. Church leaders consider seeking medical treatment as a lack of faith. Their faith-healing belief comes from the Book of James in the King James version of the Bible, where the biblical statement "the prayer of faith shall save the sick" is taken literally. Between 1955 and 1998, a total of 78 children reportedly died in Oregon City as a result of these faith-healing practices (Crombie, 2019). According to Crombie (2019), because of "the church's long history of child deaths, the Oregon Legislature in 2011 removed spiritual treatment as a defense for all homicide charges" (para 8).

In Idaho there is a cemetery that has 600 children whose families were members of the Followers of Christ Church. The deaths were a result of preventable illnesses such as pneumonia and food poisoning (Del Buono, 2016).

According to Del Buono (2016):

> It is questionable as to how members of these churches and religious denominations have legally been able to withhold medical treatment for their children and only heal through spiritual means. The First Amendment right to religious freedom, however, has given these members the ability to

practice faith healing through religious exemption laws. (p. 454)

Although the First Amendment has been interpreted to forbid government interference from restraining religious beliefs and practices, it also has been interpreted to limit religious acts. In another perspective, faith-healing affirmative defenses essentially allow for faith healers to escape criminal liability. (p. 480)

According to CHILD USA (2020) and Idahochildren.org (2020), most states continue to offer some level of parental exemption from legal prosecution when medical care is withheld from children due to religious faith. Nine states continue to have exemptions protecting parents from prosecution when their child dies from implementing their faith. Seven states have no religious exemptions from either civil or criminal charges. Twenty-one states have no exemptions for legal protection from religion-based criminal charges (see Table 7.1).

According to Swan, it appears that faith healing is declining nationwide (Green, 2019). According to Ruth Brown (2020) as stated in the *Idaho Statesman*, 13 children have died in the last five years from the application of religious faith in lieu of medical care in the state of Idaho. These deaths were attributed to heart defects, pneumonia, infection, seizures, and sepsis. In some cases, as stated by coroners' reports, the mothers received no prenatal care. To this date, exemptions continue in Idaho that protect parents from prosecution if they decline traditional medical care and apply their religious faiths and doctrines. According to Brown (2020), "Members of the Followers of Christ, a small Christian faith . . . have repeatedly told lawmakers they believe pharmaceuticals are the product of Satan, and if they give their child such products, the child will not be able to find eternity in the afterlife. Seeking any medical assistance would be contrary to their religious beliefs" (para. 21).

9 OVERVIEW OF RELIGIOUS DOCTRINES

In an article by Green (2018), a young couple, both Followers of Christ in the state of Oregon, who lost a premature infant twin born at 32 weeks during a home birth, were sentenced to prison for pleading guilty to "criminally negligent homicide and first-degree criminal mistreatment" (para. 55). In addition, approximately two dozen children of Oregon's Followers of Christ Church members have died since the 1950s due to the absence of seeking medical care that was needed to survive what was considered to be treatable conditions ranging from pneumonia to a urinary tract obstruction (Green, 2018).

CHAPTER 10

THE IMPORTANCE OF CULTURAL COMPETENCE

Race, ethnicity, and culture are three terms often misused in our healthcare system. The term *culture* is distinctly different, as a cultural group can represent several races and even ethnicities. According to Lipson, Dibble, and Minarik (1996), "The people of the world can be seen as a tapestry woven of many different strands. Those strands are integral to the whole, yet each retains an individuality that enriches the beauty of the cloth" (p. iv). The cloth can be seen as cultural diversity, the strands as what each individual brings to the tapestry.

According to Lipson et al. (1996), "It is also important to understand and respect the healthcare culture within which the nurse is practicing. That culture, whether located within the hospital, home and/or community, is influenced by intersections of forces larger than the individual" (p. iv). Cultural norms are taught by many influencing factors. Individuals, such as cultural leaders, elders within a community, or even clergy, can be highly influential in creating cultural norms.

Small groups within a larger cultural group also may influence what are considered to be acceptable behaviors or beliefs.

Similar to religious groups, not all members of every cultural group adopt the cultural norms that may influence adults or parents' healthcare decisions. Not all Muslims may subscribe to cultural norms pertaining to diet and lifestyle. Not all Jews aspire to religious norms required of faith-based Jewish members. Not all Hindus refuse beef-based medications and diets. Values seen within a cultural group may not be considered applicable to all group members. Autonomy, for example, may be highly valued by some members of a cultural group and not by others. Healthcare professionals should ask what cultural preferences are important and seek reasonable and accessible alternatives.

Resources on Cultural Diversity in Pediatric and Adult Healthcare

Leininger, M., & McFarland, M. (2002). *Transcultural nursing: Concepts, theories, research and practice* (3rd ed.). McGraw-Hill.

Linnard-Palmer, L., & Kools, S. (2004). Parents' refusal of medical treatment based on religious and/or cultural beliefs: The law, ethical principles, and clinical implications. *Journal of Pediatric Nursing, 19*(5), 351–356.

Lipson, J., Dibble, S., & Minarik, P. (1996). *Culture and nursing care: A pocket guide.* UCSF Nursing Press.

Rosaldo, R. (1993). *Culture and truth: The remaking of social analysis* (2nd ed.). Beacon.

10   THE IMPORTANCE OF CULTURAL COMPETENCE

According to Sattar et al. (2004), there are over 1,000 pharmaceutical products made from animal products whose use may go against cultural and/or religious beliefs, creating what has been called an "ethical conflict." According to their research study, 70% of physicians surveyed were reported to be unaware of medications that contain components that could be seen as being against one's religion, and 63% of patients surveyed reported that they wanted their caregivers to provide information on medications that could be against religious or cultural beliefs. Research has shown that physicians, in general, attempt to navigate tension, respect autonomy, and provide flexibility yet try to persuade medical recommendations (Curlin et al., 2005). Table 10.1 includes examples of these animal-based products.

Table 10.1 Examples of Animal-Based Pharmaceuticals: Porcine (Pig), Bovine (Cow), Equine (Horse), and Murine (Mouse)

Animal Product	Pharmaceutical Products Used In
Porcine	Clexane: enoxaparin anticoagulant, anti-thrombotics
	Creon: pancrelipase digestive supplement and cholelitholytic
	Heparin sodium injection and heparinized saline: anticoagulant
	Rotarix: live attenuated human rotavirus vaccine
	Orgaran: hemostatic agent (danaparoid) from animal mucosa

continues

Table 10.1 Examples of Animal-Based Pharmaceuticals: Porcine (Pig), Bovine (Cow), Equine (Horse), and Murine (Mouse) (cont.)

Animal Product	Pharmaceutical Products Used In
Bovine	Cartilage: anti-inflammatory and analgesic
	Ethical Nutrients Inner Health Plus Power: bovine colostrum digestive lactobacillus supplement
	Haemacel: plasma volume expander
	Hypurin isophane (NPH): insulin preparation
	Tisseel VH S/D solution: factor XIII-fibrinogen, calcium chloride dehydrate-thrombin hemostatic agent
	Travelan: bovine colostrum antidiarrheal medication
	Virivax: live varicella zoster vaccine
	Vivaxim: salmonella typhi vaccine and hepatitis A vaccine
	Zypast collagen implants: collagen dermatological preparation
Equine	Antivenom for the black, brown, and death adder
	Premarin tablets: conjugated oestrogens gonadal hormone
	Premia: medroxyprogesterone acetate gonadal hormone
	Red black spider antivenom
	Antivenom for sea snake, stonefish, and taipan
Murine	Avastin bevacizumab antineoplastic agent
	Remicade: immunomodifier/monoclonal antibody
	Saizen: pituitary hormone

(Curlin et al., 2005; Queensland Health, 2013; Sattar et al., 2004)

… THE IMPORTANCE OF CULTURAL COMPETENCE

THEORETICAL INFLUENCES: DECISION-MAKING MODELS

The use of theory is beneficial in the interpretation of complex phenomena. Theory allows members of health science professionals to view concepts and constructs as a way to make sense of, or make clear, elements of human response that are multifaceted. Ethical dilemmas have long been studied with the assistance of theoretical explanations.

Talking about the value of life when discussing the withholding of medical treatment can shed light on a parent's decision to refuse or withhold treatment. If parents' religious or cultural convictions are so strong they compel a conscious decision to apply the doctrine rather than sustain the life of their child, then viewing the value of the child's life becomes unclear. *Vitalism*—the doctrine that "vital forces" are active in living organisms, so that life cannot be explained solely by mechanism—as discussed by Paris (1982), is that theoretical construct that provides a perspective on the value of life: "Life is the ultimate value, and something that is to be preserved regardless of prognosis, regardless of cost, and regardless of social considerations" (p. 121). In contrast, parents with powerful religious convictions believe the application of religious law is by far more important than preserving life. An interview with a Jehovah's Witness nurse supports this conviction:

> My relationship with God is paramount. My desire to ascend to His house is all encompassing to me. I would not, under any circumstances, ever, allow a blood transfusion to enter my veins, as this is God's law. It is clearly written in the Bible over and over . . . you will not take blood into the body as blood is the very soul of life. I would not allow this law to be broken even in the situation where a physician tries to explain to me the need. No. Not ever. I love

my God, and He loves me. I follow his word and his rules. (personal communication, spring 2000)

According to Paris (1982, p. 144):

> We should always proceed with humility, with caution, with tentativeness, with a tilt to the side of life; with the understanding there is no such thing as life without value, that all life is valued as a gift of God and is precious in His eyes and hence, sacred for us; that whatever decision we make should be in the best interest of the child and not based on functional utility.

A standardized model for decision-making related to parents' or adults' decision to limit, delay, or refuse medical treatments is not in the current literature. Kopelman, Irons, and Kopelman (1988); Tierney, Weinberger, Greene, and Studdard (1984); Paris (1982); and Prager and Rubin (2018) have all posed concerns about the lack of a standardized process to help guide refusal scenarios. Concerns include:

- Who should be included in the decision-making process? Courts? Physicians? Solely the parents?

- How should the medico-legal and management problems of treatment refusal be handled? Who should become involved in hospital, clinic, or emergency care settings to guide the team and the process?

- What do we really have? Principles? Physician recommendations? Ad hoc decisions that can be made well or poorly?

- With no standardized or universal set of published guidelines on medical treatment refusal (beyond ways to determine decision capacity) and physician decision-making, at what point should an ethics committee consult take place?

- How do ethical principles apply, and what types of ethical decision-making processes really fit?

10 THE IMPORTANCE OF CULTURAL COMPETENCE

As stated quite clearly by Selde (2015):

> Informed refusal applies the concepts of informed consent to refusal of care. It's similar in that informed refusal seeks to best respect the decisions of the patient while balancing the provider's duty to care for the patient. Both of these ethical theories are complex and not completely agreed upon by experts in their overall application . . . The first step in the process of informed refusal is to establish if the patient is their own medical decision-maker. This relates to competence. Competence is a legal definition and is determined by a judge . . . (para 10)
>
> Once decision-maker status has been established, capacity must be determined. Unlike competence, capacity isn't a permanent state. Capacity is a patient's ability to understand their medical situation and make an informed decision about care after being advised of the risks and benefits of a particular course of action. Its existence or lack of existence can be variable. Capacity goes beyond just being alert and oriented. However, a patient who isn't alert and oriented can't have capacity. Nor can a patient who is psychotic, suicidal, or homicidal have capacity. (para. 16)

DECISION-MAKING MODELS

When seeking decision-making from the courts on treatment decisions, do jury members, or solely judges, consider both the quality of life of the child as well as the probability of recovery based on the feasibility of the treatments? Do decisions that make good sense to a judge make sound sense for the patient and the family? Who takes into account the religious doctrines that family members may hold so dear? Long-term consequences of refusal episodes to the children involved have not been investigated, and minimal references to long-term consequences to the family as a unit can be found.

Jon Watchko (1983) investigated the impact of decision-making for infants who are critically ill requiring treatment decisions. He published a theoretical discussion on a "two schools of thought model" (found to be untitled): Should the responsibility of decision-making for critically ill infants fall to the hands of a forum (committee or courts) or should it fall to the hands of the parent and physician? Watchko (1983) proposed two questions:

1. Who should participate in this decision-making process?
2. With regard to individual participants, what degree of input should be expected and invited?

If these same questions raised by Watchko were posed about a religious family in crisis concerning who will make decisions about their child, research questions could be elaborated and restated as:

1. When faith crosses paths with children's health, who should participate in the treatment decisions?
2. With regard to individual participants, such as clergy, church leaders and liaisons, family members, nurses, and physicians, how much information about one's faith should be invited as input?

Norman Fost, quoted in Watchko, within a foundational and historical context, encourages placing the decision-making responsibility on a forum (committee or courts). He argues that one action can be considered right if it would be approved by one ideal observer with these five qualities (1983, p. 795):

1. Omniscience (access to all relevant facts)
2. Omnipercipience (ability to imagine the feelings of others vividly)
3. Disinterest (having no vested interest in the situational outcomes)

4. Dispassion (keeping one's emotions in check so as not to cloud one's critical thinking)
5. Consistency, as similar cases should be decided similarly

The problem is that the ideal situation rarely arises. More often, group consensus is reached with high hopes that as much information as possible was gathered and considered with each individual case of medical care refusal. A format of the committee would include membership from a multitude of professional disciplines: nursing, clergy, social services, medical-legal, and lay public. Fost (1981) further describes the concept of "ideal observer" as the one providing the platform for the decision-making process. One may argue that, when discussing the application of one's deeply rooted faith, the notion of being an "observer" rather than one much more involved may be questionable. Fost describes how the greater the impartiality, the less chance "uncontested perception and self-interest of one party" will occur (Watchko, 1983, p. 795).

Another perspective in this first school of thought is the logical moral reasoning perspective provided by a multidisciplinary forum that places the preservation of life as of paramount importance. The conflict experienced by a parent or family desiring to follow the doctrine of their faith may surface when, like Jehovah Witnesses believe, a medical intervention would possibly condemn the child's soul (Watchko, 1983). This powerful outcome has the potential to alter the relationship between parent and child.

The second school of thought places the parental input as the vital theme. A pediatrician quoted in Watchko (1983), Dr. S. Duff, suggests that the service to families whose aim is to allow them to "evaluate largely on their own terms" (p. 796) would benefit from the input of the family members views, contributions, and adaptations. He calls this process "modified egalitarianism." Proponents of the second school of thought see this as placing the burdens of decision-making on the family because they are most familiar with the respective situation.

In previous literature, authors have proposed the notion that most parents actually use a committee, a "jury" if you will, to test the choices they plan to make or have made. This jury is made up of intimate friends, family members, clergymen, neighbors, fellow parishioners, and so on. This inherent jury already offers its views and support to the family. Families may or may not be consciously aware of their use of this inherent jury.

The final decision-making force may actually be made up of four assumptions:

1. The parents represent the non-institutional perspective of the family and child; as such, they are subjected to review by family members and pressure from various agencies, including the church and close friends.

2. The physician, even though he may be sympathetically engaged with the patient and family, primarily represents an institutional viewpoint and, as such, is subject to the constraints of peer review and pressure from other medical personnel, including nurses, social workers, and hospital administrators.

3. Hospital-based committees (interdisciplinary) would serve as consultants and advisors only, without authority to implement their decisions.

4. The courts, once involved in the decision-making process, would assume primary authority.

EMOTIONAL REACTIONS AND MORAL DISTRESS IN REFUSAL SCENARIOS

The refusal of medical treatments for children is a highly complex phenomenon that can create profound emotional reactions for both healthcare professionals and families. Emotional reactions can include fear, anguish, stress, anxiety, grief, tension, anger, and guilt. Although limited research has been conducted in the past on the impact of refusal episodes on those involved, the results of the authors' ethnographic inquiry is presented in Chapter 12, shedding light on how influential these powerful ethical dilemmas are on those involved. For now, a discussion will follow about how previous researchers and authors have described the impact of refusal scenarios on emotional well-being.

The nearby sidebar lists families' and healthcare professionals' responses to scenarios of refusal or limitation of medical treatment, with or without the loss of guardianship, demonstrating the variations of a single theme: that refusal situations are indeed emotionally charged.

Common Responses to Refusal or Limitation of Medical Treatment

- Families experience grief compounded by a report and investigation of possible medical neglect of their children. (Kopelman et al., 1988)

- Families of Jehovah's Witnesses may feel confused, stress loss of control, feel guilt, and perhaps some relief that the decision (transfusion therapy) is not, or is no longer, theirs to make. (Anderson, 1983)

- Forced treatment on competent patients comes via "forceful persuasion." Guilt may appear in relation to patient's fears of having embarrassed the physician. Guilt may appear in having expressed anger. (Appelbaum & Roth, 1983)

- The result of the violation of a deeply held, longstanding religious conviction can be devastating. (Fox, 1990)

- Those who hold religious beliefs that conflict with mainstream medical practice create tension for clinicians between honoring the different religious perspectives of the individual or carrying out what they believe to be their professional obligations. (Lawry et al., 1996)

- The stress nurses experience when involved with treatment decisions for Jehovah's Witnesses is discussed by Thurkauf (1989). Nurses are encouraged to verbalize their feelings, both to each other or as a group.

- "Dilemmas are particularly complex when the patient involved is a child, not only because of the emotional nature of the situation, but also because of the uncertainty about who has moral and legal responsibility for authorization of treatment or withholding treatment." (Overbay, 1996, p. 19)

- The concepts of "moral force" and "bilateral perceptions of being right" as discussed by Foreman (1999) concerned the professional/parent argument over decision-making around a child's medical treatment.

- Forum advocates, such as in ethics committees and courts, describe reactions by parents such as denial, fear, anger, and guilt at the time when critical decisions may need to be made. (Watchko, 1983)

- Refusal or postponement of medical care can result in what is considered tension within three values of society: 1) responsibility of parents; 2) freedom of religion; and 3) the societal responsibility of protecting children. (Orr, 2003)

A quote that clearly summarizes suggestions for clinical practice offered by Orr (2003, para. 9) is:

> When parents hold a religious belief that leads them to refuse treatment for a child, at least 2 levels of under-

standing are needed in an effort to reach agreement. The parents need to understand the clinical situation as clearly as possible. This may sometimes be facilitated or augmented by obtaining a second (or third) opinion. It is ethically permissible to try to persuade the parents using honest facts and clear opinions, though it could be perceived as harassment if attempts at persuasion are frequent or authoritarian.

In addition, the healthcare professionals need to understand the religious belief as clearly as possible. These beliefs may sometimes be well understood and clearly articulated by the parents. It is often helpful, however, to involve a 'religious translator' in the conversation, i.e., a chaplain or perhaps another person from the parents' own faith tradition, and preferably a person with some depth of education and position of authority. One reason for utilizing such a resource person is that parents (or anyone) may sometimes focus on one religious tenet while ignoring a balancing tenet; e.g., waiting for a miracle versus an obligation to preserve life and relieve suffering. A more objective look at the entire faith tradition may sometimes allow parents the freedom to consent to procedures without feeling they have abandoned the teachings of their faith.

MORAL DISTRESS

Moral distress, as a concept, has had much attention in the health sciences literature. Moral distress has been defined as an emotional reaction one has toward emotionally painful or emotionally distressing situations. As medical technology evolves, as families represent unique cultural groups, as more and more ethical dilemmas arise, and as legal interventions continue to highly influence medicine, moral distress for healthcare professionals will continue to grow. Needless to say, individuals, families, and groups all can experience moral distress as the involvement in complex ethical dilemmas reaches beyond the patient themselves.

Moral distress has been described in several ways:

- Examples of moral distress shared in pediatric nursing literature include powerful reflections of unresolved emotions and unresolved emotional conflicts with the families or doctors. Some nurses report that moral distress is the outcome of unresolved conflicts (personal communication, pediatric nursing research focus group, 2003). Very little literature is found on this topic.

- Moral distress can be defined and described as a complex experience lacking a complete definition but increasing in frequency. One factor in the development and experience of moral distress is that of technological advancements influencing the experience of life and death decisions and as being a part of healthcare occupational issues (Hanna, 2004).

- Moral distress is identified as having three types: shocked, muted, and chronic (dormant and unresolved) (Hanna & Roy, 2001).

- Moral distress may occur when nurses are unable to translate their moral choices into moral action, not being included in the decision-making (Perkin et al., 1997).

- In moral distress, a nurse knows the morally right course of action to take but institutional structures and conflicts with co-workers create obstacles (Jameton, 1993).

- In relation to the COVID-19 pandemic, "Moral distress is well described amongst HCWs and leads to stress, burnout, and lack of resilience. We would thus emphasize the cumulative emotional toll that follows having to navigate frequent, and often nebulous, ethical dilemmas at the frontlines of the pandemic" (Veins et al., 2020, para. 1).

The following describes moral distress in relation to participation in ethical dilemmas:

- The professional role one plays leads to differences in moral action, not so much differences in ethical reasoning or moral motivation (Corley et al., 2001).
- The Moral Distress Scale (Corley et al., 2001) has 32 items on a 7-point Likert scale. A factor analysis yielded three variations of moral distress: individual responsibility, not in the patient's best interest, and deception.
- Moral distress was found to be associated with anger and frustration, leading to burnout of experienced nurses (Sundin-Huard & Fahy, 1999).
- Moral distress was found to be associated with the inability to translate moral choices into moral action (Perkin et al., 1997).

How one copes with moral distress may be quite unique. Some people may carry moral distress with them for a length of time, compounded with each new morally distressing situation, leading them to leave professional practice. Others may be far more able to adjust with each "dose" of moral distress and carry on with strength.

CHAPTER 11

PROFESSIONAL GROUPS' REACTIONS TO TREATMENT REFUSAL: NURSING, MEDICINE, RESEARCHERS, AND JOURNALISTS

Health science professionals and those in related disciplines frequently hold membership in one or more of a variety of professional organizations. Nursing and medicine, for example, have literally dozens of professional organizations that represent the variety of disciplines or paths people may take in their professional career. Some of these organizations take stances on politically charged social issues, while others limit their social policy work and specialize in educational and professional development. After reviewing the literature for position papers, suggestions, or opinions on the phenomenon of treatment refusal or limitation for children based on their parents' religious beliefs, only seven were found. The following discussion will disclose a variety of perspectives of professional groups. These discussions center on the professional perspectives of how influential parents are on the healthcare decisions for children.

NURSING

No nursing organization has published a position paper expressing views on this subject, and very few published articles specially written to guide nurses in their roles, responsibilities, legal perspectives, or clinical standards on the topic of treatment refusal could be located. Upon questioning nurse executives, nurse leaders, and directors of hospital operations on the subject of treatment refusal, no standardized policies, procedures, or clinical guidelines could be located by these professionals.

Members of the Christian Nursing Society, California chapter, have communicated their stance on medical treatment refusal or limitation via informal interviews in 2000. Although members of this professional organization hold a variety of job classifications (some in pediatrics, most in care of adults), their mission statement was described as *upholding and practicing Christian principles in their professional practices*. The society has published the position that *it is right to not only explain that Jehovah's Witnesses' (JW) interpretation of the Bible is incorrect, but also that it is justified to attempt to talk a JW parent out of their transfusion refusal*. This was a sentence found in the literature, not a complete position paper. This intolerance of diverse views may limit and harm the therapeutic relationship needed between a professional nurse and JW family members.

11 PROFESSIONAL GROUPS' REACTIONS TO TREATMENT REFUSAL

At the time of this writing, this topic has been presented to 13 different professional organizations. At each of the sessions, whether a podium or a poster presentation, dozens of nurses acknowledged the complexity of the topic and shared their personal experiences. Many of the nurses expressed concern not only for the well-being of the child but also for the growing number of treatment refusal situations they have encountered as practicing nurses. The overarching theme found in these informal discussions was that there simply is not enough information available to guide their practice and help them through these ethical dilemmas or assist them with long-term feelings of moral distress.

PHYSICIANS

Quotes from several physicians have demonstrated strong opposition to religious influence on treatment decisions. For example, Foreman (1999) states that "conflicts between caretakers and practitioners can arise when families are reckless in making decisions about their children, and when families hold views that are incompatible with the treatment offered" (p. 464). The use of the term *reckless* connotates strong sentiment.

The American Academy of Pediatrics (AAP) Committee on Bioethics published guidelines back in 1988 on religious exemptions from child abuse. The following is an opening quote:

> Children sometimes die or become disabled when they fail to receive medical treatment because of the strongly held religious or philosophical beliefs or practices of their parents. The numbers of such incidents of neglect are hard to ascertain reliably, but there are increasingly frequent reports in the mass media. We believe that the reported cases represent a much larger problem. (p. 169)

AGAINST MEDICAL ADVICE

The AAP Committee on Bioethics (1988, pp. 170–171) offers guidelines, stating:

> The American Academy of Pediatrics recommends that all pediatricians, pediatric surgeons, and AAP state chapters vigorously take the lead to: (1) increase public awareness of the hazards to children growing out of religious exemptions to child abuse and neglect legislation; (2) support legislation in each state legislature to correct statutes and regulations that permit harm to children under the shield of religious exemptions; (3) work with other child advocacy organizations and agencies to develop coordinated and concerted public and professional actions for revision of religious exemptions. The academy must unequivocally defend the rights of all children to the protection and benefits of the law and medicine when physical harm—or life itself—is in the balance.

Another pertinent quote from the AAP (1988, p. 170) states:

> The Committee on Bioethics asserts: (1) the opportunity to grow and develop safe from physical harm with the protection of our society is a fundamental right of every child; (2) the basic moral principles of justice and of protection of children as vulnerable citizens require that all parents and caretakers must be treated equally by the laws and regulations that have been enacted by state and federal governments to protect children; (3) all child abuse, neglect, and medical neglect statutes should be applied without potential or actual exemption for religious beliefs; (4) no statute should exist that permits or implies that denial of medical care necessary to prevent death or serious impairment to children can be supported on religious grounds; (5) state legislatures and regulatory agencies with interests in children should be urged to remove religious exemptions clauses from statutes and regulations.

11 PROFESSIONAL GROUPS' REACTIONS TO TREATMENT REFUSAL

Updated guidelines published in 1997 by the American Academy of Pediatrics' Committee on Bioethics describe how exemptions to child neglect and child abuse laws continue to restrict the ability to protect children by limiting government actions or the seeking of legal redress when alleged neglect or abuse occurs in the name of religion. AAP guidelines are that legal intervention should apply equally every time a child is harmed without the acceptance of religious faith exemptions. AAP continues to call for the repeal of religious exemption laws (AAP Committee on Bioethics, 1997).

Dr. Seth Asser, as quoted to *Time* magazine's David Van Biema (Reaves, 2001, p. 1), stated:

> Kids die from accidental deployment of air bags, and you get hearings in Congress. But this goes on (child deaths or injury from parents' refusal of medical care), and dozens die, and people think there's no problem because the deaths happen one at a time. But the kids who die suffer horribly. This is Jonestown in slow motion.

PROFESSIONAL JOURNALISTS: CURRENT AND HISTORICAL PERSPECTIVES

Journalists have demonstrated an ongoing interest in locating and following the outcomes of pediatric medical treatment refusals. Although sometimes the articles may be interpreted as sensationalized, journalist investigation has been shown to be fruitful in uncovering cases of neglect, abuse, and treatment refusal, as well as subsequent prosecution, acquittal, and other related legal consequences.

According to Wilson (2016), a journalist from the Guardian in Boise, Idaho, parents of religious organizations that refuse or limit healthcare continue to have legal protection that Wilson titled, "a faith-based shield from felony crimes such as manslaughter" (para. 5). Wilson gives a historical perspective stating that the "shield laws" protecting parents are "an artifact of the Nixon administration" (para. 6) when high-profile cases led activists to encourage the creation of laws to protect children from harm including the Child Abuse Prevention and Treatment Act (CAPTA) signed by Nixon in 1974. At that time, two presidential advisors, J.R. Haldeman and John Ehrlichman, both jailed for their role in the Watergate scandal, and both members of a faith-healing sect, influenced the creation of the laws with a provision allowing those who only participate in prayer for healing to benefit from an exception. Over time, the federal laws changed but some states continue to have laws supporting the exception. Even to this day, religious liberty is a powerfully debated topic.

Michael Rubinkam, a journalist from Pennsylvania wrote a piece (updated February 2, 2017) concerning Pennsylvania parents who implemented their religious faith healing in lieu of taking their 2-year-old daughter for medical care for pneumonia. She died at home. Released on bail and home with their other six children, the parents, members of Faith Tabernacle Church, vowed to take their other children to see medical professionals in the future. Pennsylvania authorities say future cases would be prosecuted.

In 1985, Denise Houseman was taken by her older brother to a local hospital in Pennsylvania to be admitted to the ICU for severe complications of Crohn's disease. The family, active members in a Faith Tabernacle church, did not seek any medical care for their daughter as their faith not only forbade it, but considered disease to be a "moral issue, the result of being out of relationship with God" (para. 3). Now an adult with a family, Mrs. Houseman is not a part of the religious sect and states, the members of the church "are not monsters" rather "they are hardworking… responsible…who don't know any better" (para. 20). According to journalist DeJesus, "Trying to convince legislatures to repeal religious exemptions remains a perennial battle for advocates, particularly amid the growing tide of conservative legislatures that favor religious freedoms" (para. 69).

11 PROFESSIONAL GROUPS' REACTIONS TO TREATMENT REFUSAL

Joel Dyer, a writer for Colorado's *Boulder Weekly*, has done extensive research on the topic of parents' refusal of medical care for religious preferences. He has studied both cults and well-established churches in America. He wrote his opinions on Colorado House Bill 1286, passed by the Colorado House of Representatives, which mandates criminal prosecution of people who withhold medical treatment from a seriously ill child. He describes this in his article "Faith Healing and Dying Kids" (www.boulderweekly.com, 2000, para. 6):

> I have to report that, as a rule, people like Amanda's parents (who prayed for their dying daughter instead of seeking medical care) actually love their children just as much as the rest of us love ours. They mourn the loss of children with equally sincere passion. People in faith-healing cults do what they do because they love their children, not because they are monsters. For a number of reasons, including what amounts to being brainwashed by a cult, faith healing adherents . . . are truly convinced that avoiding medical care is the best thing they can do for their kids. As much as we don't want to believe it is true, these people have no easier time watching their children die than the rest of us do.

Dyer (2000, para. 7) wrote that the law will likely not make much of a difference. He believes:

> The new law will not save a single child's life. Can we really expect people who have been brainwashed to the extent that they are willing to let the baby they love bleed to death in their arms from a simple wound to suddenly be motivated to seek medical care because they fear being charged with a crime? It's not likely. All this new law will accomplish is to put a small handful of grieving, misguided, brainwashed parents into prison and further radicalize and isolate the faith-healing cults that are actually responsible for the parent's contaminated thinking. And further

isolating these cults will only make it more unlikely that deaths such as Amanda's will be prevented or even discovered.

Dyer (2000) further describes how many of these organizations exist on the fringes of society, encouraging parents to homeschool their children, thus making it even more difficult to locate and report these families to authorities. Dyer believes a bill like this will actually cause more children's deaths rather than stopping them, as those parents who have historically rushed their children to EDs and hospitals for last-minute interventions will now fear prosecution.

Mark Larabee, a journalist for *The Oregonian*, wrote an article titled "The Battle Over Faith Healing: When Prayer Pre-empts Medical Care: Prosecutor's Nationwide Struggle to Respect Parents' Freedoms While Protecting Children's Lives" (November 28, 1998). His article describes cases where children have lost their lives from such medical conditions as diabetes, Wilms tumor, cystic fibrosis, stomach cancer, and complications from prematurity, home births, and labor trauma while their parents hold on to their religious convictions against seeking traditional medical care. The article gives an interesting discussion of the defending lawyer for faithful parents, citing that one lawyer stated (Larabee, 1998, as quoted by attorney Arthur Jarrett, p. 4):

> Loving parents shouldn't be prosecuted for doing what they think is best for their children. It's not neglect if you actually believe it and you do what your religion says to do to get healed and you do it fervently. You can't prosecute religion away. It does not alter the religious practice. Outside of venting a public desire, it furthers no interest.

Journalist David Kostinchuk (2001) poses interesting questions in his article "Faith Healing: Child Abuse, Torture and Homicide." He asks the question, "Can faith healing be likened to torture?" He describes how the right to refuse medical treatment based on religious grounds is well supported by many societies when the individual is a consenting adult. But what happens when the person is a child? Kostinchuk

11 PROFESSIONAL GROUPS' REACTIONS TO TREATMENT REFUSAL

(2001) states that the child of this phenomenon will most likely suffer "for very abstract reasons, which in all likelihood he or she does not understand" (p. 1). His expressed opinion is that this is not torture, but rather, at least, an extreme form of child abuse.

There is no single, overarching theme developed by pediatric healthcare professionals to guide the practitioner through refusal scenarios. Nurses, physicians, and journalists vary on their views of pediatric treatment refusal, be it torture, child abuse, child neglect, religious brainwashing, group normative behaviors, misguided or misled behaviors, or simply faithful parents with distinct methods of conduct. It is quite justifiable for professional groups like the Society of Pediatric Nurses or the American Academy of Pediatrics to publish clinical practice guidelines.

Journalists Foy and Pfannenstiel (2018) describe the perspective of legal officials who encounter child deaths from faith healing and their frustration with the dichotomy of religious freedom versus protecting vulnerable children. For instance, in Canyon County, Idaho, Coroner Vicki DeGeus-Morris, who lost a primary election to the former Deputy Coroner Jennifer Crawford, has often been the first official to investigate deaths in Canyon County related to faith healing. She received criticism for her role in reporting child deaths that surfaced during her campaign. Crawford stated in the article that "The Followers of Christ have been totally cooperative, and I have never had any problems with them," and, "I don't judge. It's not my place to judge them. The Legislature has to change that law" (Foy & Pfannenstiel, 2018, para. 16). Foy and Pfannenstiel (2018) describe how "Activists say repealing faith-healing protections is a matter of helping children who can't help themselves, while the faith-healing community claims the heart of the debate lies in protecting religious freedom" (para. 7).

As reported by journalist Herrskink (2020), a panel of child-welfare advocates, police, state legislators, and a former Supreme Court Chief Justice fought to change or repeal bills on exemptions of legal prosecution for parents who turn to faith healing rather than allopathic medical care and whose children have died. Repeals or changes in bills have either died in committee or have been voted down. A new bill proposed in 2020 by the group would amend Idaho's religious exemptions, and the group hopes to secure the support from the House and Senate Judiciary Committees in order to pass timely legislation.

CHAPTER 12

OVERVIEW OF PROFESSIONAL INTERVENTIONS: POWER DISTANCE, NEGOTIATION, AND SAFETY

Working with families and individuals who refuse medical treatment and vaccines requires a type of teamwork that is goal-oriented and provides safety while assessing concerns, beliefs, doctrines, and thought processing. The team working with the family must determine how to evaluate the sincerity of the treatment refusal and then determine if there are alternatives to the treatment, and if not, determine if there will be health consequences to the refusal.

Adults who refuse lifesaving medical treatments can be granted their wishes, even if the refusal ends with disability or death. Parents of minors cannot place the child in a situation where clinical outcomes are poor. Providing information on poor health outcomes may be challenging, as the information may not be accepted, even when communicated with clarity around the consequences. If the physician or primary provider is not successful in obtaining consent, *power distance* may be used to try to change the parents' or the guardian's mind. According to Hofstede (1985), a Dutch psychologist, power distance is the recognition that a perception of inequality exists between people, and that power distance can be used to influence the outcome of a debate, conversation, businesses interactions, and overall, human interactions.

According to Rutledge (2011):

> Power distance refers to the way in which power is distributed and the extent to which the less powerful accept that power is distributed unequally. Put simply, people in some cultures accept a higher degree of unequally distributed power than do people in other cultures. When in a high-power distance culture, the relationship between bosses and subordinates is one of dependence. When in a low power distance society, the relationship between bosses and subordinates is one of interdependence. (para. 1)

The Power Distance Index "refers to the degree of inequality that exists—and is accepted—between people with and without power" (Mindtools.com, n.d., para. 8). "A high PDI score indicates that a society accepts an unequal, hierarchical distribution of power, and that people understand 'their place' in the system. A low PDI score means that power is shared and is widely dispersed, and that society members do not accept situations where power is distributed unequally" (Mindtools.com, n.d., para. 9).

In healthcare settings, power distance may be used with those who feel less powerful, causing them to speak out less about their perceptions, needs, and wants. According to Whisenant (2019), power distance within the healthcare arena is one of two professions that have historically had negative effects (the other is aviation). With power distance, patients and their families may not speak up, defend their beliefs, or even seek guidance or treatment from those they feel have more power over them. Those who have deeply held religious, cultural, or philosophical beliefs may perceive power as a phenomenon that prevents them from seeking healthcare at all, as they may feel threatened, disrespected, or even dismissed.

ETHNOGRAPHIC RESEARCH IN TREATMENT REFUSAL CASES

Three research studies have been conducted by the primary author of this book (Linnard-Palmer, 2006, 2021; Linnard-Palmer & Kools, 2005) investigating how treatment refusals are experienced. This section presents three studies that can shed light on the experience: one about families who refuse medical care, one about healthcare professionals' experiences, and one that presents nurses' views of the use of power distance in healthcare when medical treatment is refused. In all three studies, the research methodology of ethnography was used as a means to study human behavior in the context of culture exchanges. According to Leininger and McFarland (2002), ethnography and ethnonursing are means to investigate how culture is experienced as biological, physical, spiritual, and historical human exchanges take place. When healthcare providers focus on cultural influences on healthcare decisions and provide culturally congruent care, personal values, beliefs, and expressions can be better understood. This results in appropriate, safe, and meaningful care.

Ethnography and enthnonursing (Lenininger & McFarland, 2002) are one way to study culture. *Culture* is a learned, adaptive, and shared way within groups of people with identifiable patterns, symbols, and material and nonmaterial data. According to Leininger and McFarland (2002), knowledge of how to provide medically safe and culturally congruent, responsible, and sensitive care is lacking. Cultural conflicts, imposition practices, stresses, and pain are the consequences of this knowledge deficit.

Ethnography is inductive, scientific, investigative, and rigorous, and emphasizes the perspectives of people in the research setting. Ethnography takes the position that behavior and the ways in which people construct and make meaning of their worlds and their lives are highly variable and locally specific (those that originate in and are found in one specific location). Ethnography assumes that one must first discover what people actually do and the reasons they give for doing it. The researcher enters as an invited guest, using self as the data collection instrument, and uses keen eyesight and hearing to discover, learn the meaning of, and steer away from any control that would influence the integrity of the local culture. The product is an interpretive story, reconstruction, or narrative about a group of people that includes their history; therefore, it paints a picture of people going about their daily lives, in the course of living out those daily lives, over a period of time. The final goal of applied ethnographic research is to understand sociocultural problems and use these understandings to bring about positive change in communities, institutions, or groups (LeCompte & Schensul, 1999).

The ethnographer assumes she must first discover what people actually do and the reasons they identify for doing things. The following are five assumptions found in the explicit definitions and goals of conducting ethnographic research:

1. Ethnography and enthnonursing seek to study culture. *Culture*—a learned, adaptive, and shared way of people with identifiable patterns, symbols, and material and nonmaterial

12 OVERVIEW OF PROFESSIONAL INTERVENTIONS

data—has biological, physical, spiritual, and historical features that healthcare providers can know and understand.

2. Culturally congruent and beneficial nursing care can only occur when healthcare values, expressions, or patterns are known and used explicitly for appropriate, safe, and meaningful care. Cultural conflicts, cultural imposition practices, cultural stresses, and cultural pain reflect the lack of culture-care knowledge needed by healthcare professionals to provide culturally congruent, responsible, safe, and sensitive care (Leininger & McFarland, 2002).

3. Culture may be defined as a system of symbols that are shared, learned, and passed on through generations of a social group. Culture links human beings and chaos—it is the basis of what people perceive and what guides people's interactions with each other. It is a process rather than a static entity, and it changes over time (Lipson et al., 1996).

4. Ethnography involves the ethnographer participating, overtly and covertly, in people's daily lives for an extended period of time, watching, listening, asking questions, and collecting data. The object is to throw light on the issues that are the focus of the research, all the time identifying the routine ways in which people make sense of the world in everyday life. The value of ethnography as a social research method is founded upon the existence of such variations in cultural patterns, across and within societies, and their significance for understanding social processes (Hammersley & Atkinson, 1993).

5. Ethnography involves an ongoing attempt to place specific encounters, events, and understandings into a fuller, more meaningful context. As a result, research design, fieldwork, and various methods of inquiry to produce historically, politically, and personally situated accounts, descriptions, interpretations, and representations of human lives are combined. Ethnography is both a process and a product. The experience is meaningful, and human behavior is generated from and

informed by this meaningfulness. The pioneers of ethnography experienced fieldwork not merely as a rite of passage, but rather the lived reality that was the center of their intellectual and emotional lives (Denzin & Lincoln, 2000).

Ethnographic methodology is an excellent fit for the investigation of cultural exchanges between healthcare providers and families whose religious, cultural, or philosophical beliefs influence healthcare decisions for children. Following are three studies for which ethnographic methodology was used to discover meaning behind cultural exchanges.

STUDY #1: PARENTAL REFUSAL OF MEDICAL TREATMENT FOR CULTURAL OR RELIGIOUS BELIEFS: AN ETHNOGRAPHIC STUDY OF HEALTHCARE PROFESSIONALS' EXPERIENCES (LINNARD-PALMER & KOOLS, 2005)

INTRODUCTION

When families refuse medical treatment for cultural or religious reasons, a variety of processes and conclusions can occur. Healthcare team members may attempt to negotiate with the family concerning treatment for acutely ill children. When negotiation of educational attempts proves unsuccessful in obtaining parental consent, healthcare professionals may request an ethics committee consultation. If the child's condition is unstable and expeditious treatments are required, the healthcare team may seek temporary legal guardianship (mandated by the state) to administer the recommended medical interventions. Not all parental treatment limitations or refusal decisions require these ethics committee or state guardianship procedures. Sometimes the parents want to have their beliefs heard and acknowledged, or they want to delay treatment so prayer sessions or cultural practices can be performed.

Ethnographic research has demonstrated that each refusal episode is unique and requires individualized considerations and actions.

METHODS

Twenty ethnographic interviews were conducted over 45 minutes to 2 hours and audio taped. Locations varied from coffee shops, classrooms, parks, and offices. Field notes were collected when appropriate. Interviews were open-coded, and themes were identified. Data were limited through the development of salient categories that grouped related concepts into broad themes. Participants revealed three types of refusal scenarios:

1. A child is brought into the healthcare arena with a medical condition directly linked to or attributed to the parents' cultural or religious-based health practices. Examples disclosed in the data: untreated communicable diseases for which immunizations were available, infections, sepsis, and diet-related cases of severe anemia.

2. A child develops a treatable medical condition that was not the consequence of the family's cultural health practices or religious beliefs, yet the family's religious or cultural belief system did not allow them to agree to curative treatment. Examples disclosed in the data include chemotherapy for early stages of retinoblastoma and blood products for severe anemia associated with vaso-occlusive episodes related to sickle cell anemia.

3. A child is brought to a physician suffering from a severe medical condition that has a dismal prognosis. The parents continue to refuse medical treatment and, at times, symptom management, even at the risk of losing guardianship to the state based on medical neglect.

FINDINGS

Three main themes emerged after careful analysis of the data transcripts:

1. **Weathering the storm of moral conflict including emotional upheaval during the refusal scenario.** The greatest storms took place when the family's religious beliefs conflicted with the nurse's spiritual or philosophical framework, or the child was at risk for severe harm from withholding treatment. The storm is created by intense dissonance between the view of the parents and the view of the caregiver.

2. **Closeness and involvement versus distance and retreat.** Participants described how they made conscious and unconscious decisions concerning their level of involvement with the families and the refusal situation. A continuum was described that ranged from jumping right in to outright refusing to care for the child and the family.

3. **Unresolved battles between the supportive and oppositional villages.** Participants described the continuing conflict, unresolved clashes, and divergent emotions generated between the healthcare team members and the family.

SUMMARY OF FINDINGS

Refusal of medical treatment will continue in the future. With increasing state-of-the-science technological advances and increasing membership in some churches, the expectation is that conflicts will continue, beliefs will clash, convictions will continue to be expressed, and ethical dilemmas will surface.

CLINICAL APPLICATION

Healthcare providers will have stronger leadership roles as they apply cultural knowledge to strained communication at the point of care. Learning more about the impact of culture and religion on healthcare decisions can increase cultural sensitivity and maintain functioning relationships.

STUDY #2: PARENTS, CLERGY, AND COMMUNITY PERSPECTIVES ON TREATMENT REFUSAL (LINNARD-PALMER, 2006)

INTRODUCTION

With increasing church membership and vast cultural diversity expanding in the nation, treatment refusal scenarios are likely to continue to increase. The moral distress that is experienced for both healthcare workers and family members has shown to have a significant negative impact on provider-family and provider-clergy relationships. A greater acknowledgment and understanding of the dynamics surrounding medical treatment refusals are warranted.

Examples of research questions posed were: What is the impact of parental religious beliefs on the interactions between family members and the healthcare team during decision-making regarding the medical treatment of the acutely ill child? What are the processes and outcomes of medical treatment refusal, including the loss of guardianship, from the perspectives of the family and clergy?

METHODS

Seventeen interviews were conducted using an ethnographic qualitative design to investigate treatment refusal or limitation of medical treatments as experienced by family members, church community members, and clergy. Individuals were sought around the greater San Francisco Bay area and beyond, based on the identified list of churches whose doctrines or teachings were found in the literature to influence decision-making. Seventeen adult participants were secured for a one-time interview with the researcher, and data were collected over the time frame of 20 weeks. After IRB approval from the University of California, San Francisco, interviews were secured with clergy leaders (three) and church members or community members whose lives had been influenced by church doctrine (14). Church affiliations represented were from Christian Science ($n = 3$), Four Square ($n = 1$), Jehovah's Witnesses ($n = 1$), and fundamentalist Christian faiths ($n = 2$). Other research participants described themselves as active members of organizations whose beliefs had a common thread of prayer in lieu of healthcare, or prayer before healthcare, or prayer along with healthcare practices ($n = 7$).

FINDINGS

Three main themes emerged from analysis of the transcribed interviews that were carefully analyzed using thematic coding procedures and narrative analysis:

1. **Proud to be a believer.** Participants disclosed their commitment to their chosen religious organization or framework and described not only what their beliefs were but also how their life was their faith ("how I eat, how I sleep, and how I live"). They also mentioned how they balanced their faith with interacting with others. Numerous experiences were offered that demonstrated how faith transected with daily life and medical/health decision-making.

2. **Wanting out.** Participants described their experiences, or their family members experiences, with leaving their faith-based organization, including various reasons why they felt compelled to leave.

3. **Mistrust versus distrust.** Here participants discussed their views on imposing beliefs on children, how clergy/elders interact with healthcare team members (particularly physicians), and how trust intersects with healthcare treatment or interventions. One participant described a complete lack of trust in modern Western medicine, stating beliefs that antibiotics are

harmful and childhood immunizations are destructive. This participant described what they used as alternative treatments (lymphatic raking, compresses, etc.)

SUMMARY OF FINDINGS

Clergy, church members, and community members whose beliefs highly influence healthcare decision-making described two ends of a spectrum: wanting to continue to adhere to their deeply held beliefs or adamantly wanting out of their previous situation, including using the terms or phrases of "regrettable," "life being ruined," and "health being negatively affected." Many described how prayer is essential and was considered a valuable tool for their health and well-being.

CLINICAL APPLICATION

Nurses, physicians, and other healthcare providers have much to learn about what is behind the relationship between religious faith, doctrines concerning traditional and nontraditional health practices, and willingness to consent for medical care and treatments for themselves and their family members, including children. Both the sample size and general geographical influences to data limited a full spectrum of perspectives and experiences. Further research is warranted that represents a greater number of faiths and locations. Data showed that no two participants described similar priorities, experiences, or desires for their family members, showing that the complexity of the topic of medical treatment refusal and faith needs further study for a greater understanding and for healthcare professionals to use sensitive and effective communication.

STUDY #3: REFUSAL OF MEDICAL TREATMENT DUE TO RELIGIOUS AND CULTURAL BELIEFS: USE OF POWER DISTANCE TO INFLUENCE OUTCOMES (LINNARD-PALMER, 2021)

INTRODUCTION

This study investigated in greater depth the communication patterns that occur when a health professional is faced with a parent or guardian who is refusing, limiting, or delaying (hesitancy) traditional Western medical care in lieu of religious, cultural, or philosophical perspectives. The phenomenon of power distance was investigated according to healthcare professionals' experience, with conversations or confrontations between family members or guardians and physicians or other primary caregivers when faced with treatment refusals. *Power distance,* a theoretical construct first described and defined by Geert Hofstede, a Dutch psychologist known for work in organizational anthropology and international management, occurs when there is a relationship in which one party has power and the other is subordinate, recognizing that power distance exists in our complex cultures. In this study, nurses and allied healthcare professionals were asked via ethnographic qualitative research methodology to describe their experiences of power distance between healthcare team members and families who are refusing traditional healthcare, diagnostics, or treatments based on their tightly held faith, cultural values and norms, or the philosophical thinking about the detriments of Western medicine.

METHODS

Twenty-three ethnographic interviews were conducted using a qualitative design that provided questions and prompts for participants to share their clinical experiences when they believed power distance was used as a method to solicit cooperation, consent, adherence, or compliance with prescribed medical care (treatment, diagnostics, etc.)

for children. Research participants were recruited using a purposive sampling method to represent clinical experts and seasoned clinicians who provide care across patient ages and developmental stages and clinical areas of practice. Research participants represented a wide range of clinical experiences via a wide range of community, industry, hospital, clinic, and home care settings, all of whom had experiences caring for children, families, and caregivers with religious, cultural, or philosophical views influencing traditional Western medicine. Research participants included members of nursing administration, research, and clinical care.

FINDINGS

Two major themes emerged from the analysis of the data via the primary researcher and a graduate nursing student:

1. **Power distance is used as a first and last resort.** Here participants provided clinical narratives of experiences where physicians and nurse practitioners used power distance as an initial means to secure cooperation, as well as a last resort when no other conversations, negotiations, education, or persuasion worked. Several of the research participants described that they felt that as the situation escalated, the primary care provider became "nervous" about potential poor clinical outcomes and used methods of power distance to communicate their concerns or knowledge of what potential outcomes could occur resulting in harm.

2. **Power distance leaves scars.** Research participants had a range of descriptions to capture the end result of using methods of power distance as a struggle to convince faithful patients or their family members. The range spanned from anger to resentment to fatigue to exasperation. When a child was involved and could not consent for their own medical care, the struggle of using types of "power" communication to get consent or cooperation for medical treatment (often expressed as

raising one's voice, stating over and over they are the expert, and threatening to leave their physician-patient/family relationship) was more difficult than expressed by those research participants who care for adult patients.

SUMMARY OF FINDINGS

Refusal of traditional medical care is a challenging phenomenon. Families whose religious or cultural beliefs/norms conflict with traditional medical care, deemed safer and necessary for positive and error-free clinical outcomes, may feel vulnerable during conversations about refusing offered treatments. When primary care providers are faced with refusals, emotions can flare, power distance or authority over others may be used, and the outcomes can result in consent and cooperation or retreat. Safety is always held in high regard, and stressful encounters during refusals have been described as emotionally exhausting, frustrating, and time-consuming.

CLINICAL APPLICATION

More research is needed on how nurses can provide support during treatment refusals based on faith and culture in order to help avoid the use of power distance. Working as a team to find smooth solutions during stressful encounters is needed so frustration and despair are avoided.

CONCLUSION

It is the hope of these authors that the preceding three research articles can shed light on the state of treatment refusals and the experiences that occur for families and healthcare professionals. Much more research is needed to fully understand the phenomenon of treatment refusal for children and adults and the short-term and long-term outcomes of experiencing unwanted medical treatments or vaccines.

Nurses, physicians, and all other allied healthcare personnel are in a unique position to offer support and understanding to individuals and families who are experiencing dilemmas related to limiting, delaying, or refusing medical care. Whenever there are issues of this kind, very often the need for improved and/or enhanced communication is at the heart of the matter. Healthcare providers must take the time to ensure that people are fully educated and clearly understand their treatment options and the ramifications of choosing one course of action over another. Think of the Health Belief Model (see Chapter 8) and reflect upon whether people truly see themselves as being at risk for a condition. Do they understand the value of their treatment plan, or do they have misconceptions about it? Do they understand the benefits of vaccines, or do they have misconceptions about them? If there are barriers to change that the individual is struggling with, remember motivational interviewing. If you lecture people on what they should be doing instead of helping them explore their *own ideas* about ways to move forward, you are doing exactly the wrong thing. Perform a cultural and spiritual assessment. In what ways can their cultural and religious beliefs be incorporated into the treatment plan? Nurses and all other allied healthcare personnel must ruthlessly stamp out and eradicate stereotyping, racism, discrimination, bigotry, ethnocentrism, and xenophobia. There is no room for them in healthcare. Every person and every life have intrinsic value and deserve the respect of being offered high-quality care in a nonjudgmental and welcoming environment.

APPENDIX A

REASONS FOR PARENTAL DECISIONS TO REFUSE MEDICAL TREATMENT

There are numerous and powerful reasons behind parental decisions to delay, limit, or refuse medical treatment. The following list of 15 reasons was condensed from health science, law, media sources, and related literature over the past 30 years:

1. Religious frameworks concerning preference for prayer instead of or prior to any traditional medical care were found nationally and internationally.

2. Religious frameworks concerning limits on interventions such as various blood and blood product transfusion therapies, specialized diet therapies, or diagnostics have been found across America.

3. Ambiguous consenting procedures by healthcare professionals seeking parental approval and signature for medical treatments, diagnostics, or other procedures can lead to refusal to sign consent forms. Often, healthcare providers try to rush the process for obtaining consent for diagnostics, treatments, transfusion, or surgeries, leading parents to refuse or

delay consent. This rush is often related to the hectic interdisciplinary schedule of pediatric hospital departments.

4. Conflicting or ambiguous sources of information on treatment decisions are not unusual. Because of the vast array of technology and clinical trials, it is not uncommon for parents to seek second or third opinions. This can delay consent or treatments.

5. Influences on the access to sophisticated medical technology can lead to fears, confusion, and delay in treatment consent.

6. Pressures during the treatment decision-making time frame can occur. Some religious or cultural practices warrant counsel by church elders, high-level church representatives, or tribal leaders, which in turn causes treatment delays.

7. Conscientious objectors to medical care or treatment exist. Some people simply do not trust or wish to apply modern, standardized medical care. Many in this category are not affiliated with any particular cultural or religious group. Some may feel that procedures are overlapping, or repeated measures are just not warranted. Sometimes they are correct and sometimes they are not. This mistrust of medical procedures may add to the confusion.

8. Use of alternative medicine modalities rather than Western medical practices has become commonplace. With the rising number of Americans who use complementary, alternative, or integrative treatments, parental desires to apply various nontraditional healing methods are escalating.

9. Parental relationships with other siblings can become strained or compromised. The sacrifice of family life (quality of life) during the demands of care for the child requiring treatment may be perceived to be too great. In other words, families may say "no" to a complex and expensive treatment (high co-payments, etc.) for one child so that the quality of life of the family as a whole is not changed or is minimally impacted.

A REASONS FOR PARENTAL DECISIONS TO REFUSE MEDICAL TREATMENT

10. Cost in dollars and loss of employment or inability to maintain employment during care for a critically ill, acutely ill, or chronically ill child can cause parents to refuse hospitalizations and/or treatments.

11. Mental capacity of parents making treatment decisions may influence consenting procedures or treatment decision-making. Illiteracy, lower health literacy levels, lower educational levels, and poor comprehension abilities can influence whether or not a parent readily consents for medical treatment (this goes for adherence or compliance with ordered treatments as well).

12. Pressures and emotional turmoil during treatment decisions may be too great.

13. Mental capabilities of children for whom treatment decisions are being made may influence parents' treatment decisions.

14. Issues concerning best interest for the child may influence consenting procedures.

15. Concerns of quality of life for the child after complex medical treatment with few known positive outcomes may influence parental decisions.

APPENDIX B

GUIDELINES FOR STAFF FACING PARENTAL REFUSAL OF PEDIATRIC VACCINES OR MEDICAL TREATMENTS

Communication is the key to successful education and adherence to vaccinations in children when parents are showing hesitancy or refusal.

Key points in communication include the following (Grimes, 2020; Linnard-Palmer & Coats, 2010).

For refusal of medical diagnostics, medical treatments, surgery, etc. (12 steps, not necessarily in order):

1. Ensure the child is safe, cared for, and under nursing or healthcare supervision at all times. Assess for changes in clinical status that may occur as a result of the child not receiving immediate nursing or medical care (such as STAT blood product transfusion or needed medical interventions).

2. Maintain respectful contact with all family members and assess frequently for any suggestion that the family may be thinking of leaving AMA.

3. Identify the primary decision-maker within the family structure and maintain a rapport.

4. Identify the child's primary caregiver(s) and notify them right away. Let the nursing supervisor know what is happening and call a social worker. If you feel threatened or worry about the safety of the child, have security personnel on notification and/or keep the police and sheriff's contact information readily available.

5. Do not use scare tactics or fear-mongering by saying you will report the family to the public health department or child protective services (make no threats).

6. Do not use your authoritative position as a healthcare professional to push the topic, as parents do not want to be told what to do, and stating or communicating you "know more than they do" will turn them off. Explain calmly the necessary treatments and/or diagnostic exams and procedures that the child requires.

7. Request the name of the family's church, organization, or cultural group whose teaching or doctrines are influencing consent or refusal to participate in medical treatment or diagnostic procedures. Look up what is needed to educate the team on the beliefs or doctrines. Identify if the organization has leaders who would need to be contacted for further information and negotiations. Ask your team's permission to ask the family for phone numbers of the clergy, elders, or contact people associated with the religion, faith, or cultural group.

8. Obtain the healthcare institution's policy and procedures for how to handle these situations. Notify the institution's administrative team. Do not talk to or contact media. Do not allow media personnel to enter the clinic or unit or get anywhere near the family. Contact security if media personnel arrive.

B GUIDELINES FOR PARENTAL REFUSAL OF MEDICAL TREATMENTS

9. Plan on coordinating a family conference with appropriate healthcare professionals.

10. Provide support and respect and keep in constant communication with family. Explain what is happening (keeping safety in mind) and why and who is involved. Be factual and straightforward, and keep explaining that your priority is the well-being of the child and family members.

11. Always document carefully with full legal perspectives in mind. It is highly likely that if the child's health or life is in danger, child protective services will become involved, and charting will be required to be submitted to official decision-makers. A lawsuit may be inevitable.

12. Attempt, when safe and possible, to include church members, faith practices, cultural practices, prayer sessions, or any safe and appropriate practices that the family may request in the plan of care. Check with the institution's supervisor if a practice is potentially unsafe or prohibited (such as candle-burning with oxygen tanks or lines close by).

For refusal, hesitancy, delay, or questioning about childhood vaccines:

1. Do not be defensive or judgmental about the parent's concerns, questions, or knowledge, as there is a lot to learn and know about childhood vaccines.

2. Do not use technical language or advanced medical terminology. Teach the family what they need to know to make safe decisions. Talk about what happens when a child receives a vaccine, as the parent may not know, such as:

    - Vaccine enters your child's body via a syringe and needle.
    - Your child's immune system will respond by creating large numbers of antibodies to the microbial substance or toxin.

- Antibodies then stand ready to fight hard against the germ when your child is exposed by attaching themselves to the germ circulating in the blood.
- Not all vaccines will give life-long immunity (fight), so boosters are required.
- Vaccines are given in specific time intervals to maximize the production of antibodies to fight disease.
- Serious childhood diseases are found all over the world and can be prevented by adhering to the recommended childhood vaccine schedule.

3. Make sure your message aligns with national and international organizations whose reputation and information sources are accessible. Provide VIS (vaccine information sheets) in the family's primary language. Print out and provide vaccination schedules.

4. Use storytelling if you have to in order to make your point.

5. Inform the primary healthcare provider for assistance in talking to and educating the family. Document carefully all that is said.

According to Gunduz et al. (2014), hospitalizations, especially for children between birth and 2 years of age, are the most commonly encountered types of pediatric healthcare refusals; therefore, clarifying reasons, overcoming deficiencies, resolving problems identified, improving conditions, and building confidence between the healthcare provider and team and the family are essential.

No matter what the refusal, delay, limitation, or hesitancy is, make sure all members of the healthcare team involved have a formal debriefing so everyone can learn and be more prepared in the future!

APPENDIX C

GUIDELINES FOR STAFF FACING ADULT REFUSAL OF MEDICAL TREATMENTS

According to Lu and Adams (2009), five basic tenets are considered foundational for informed consent associated with medical treatment refusal for adults:

1. The patient must have sufficient information about his or her medical condition.

2. The patient must understand the risks and benefits of available options, including the option not to act.

3. The patient must have the ability to use the above information to make a decision in keeping with their personal values.

4. The patient must be able to communicate their choices.

5. The patient must have the freedom of will to act without undue influence from other parties, including family and friends.

APPENDIX D

LOSS OF PARENTAL GUARDIANSHIP: COURT OVERRIDING OF A PARENT'S RIGHT TO REFUSE MEDICAL TREATMENT

WHAT IS GUARDIANSHIP?

A *guardianship* of a person is a legal process and is sometimes needed when, no matter how much parents love their child, they are not able to parent or provide for them. The appointed guardian has full legal and physical custody and can make all decisions about the child's physical needs. There are two inquiries: the parental competence (physical, emotional, and mental) and the parents' willingness to make appropriate decisions for their child, including medical care. Guardianship is based on a legal obligation by parents to refrain from actions that may harm their child. Generally, when the mental or physical health of a child is not at stake, the Supreme Court, states, and local courts will defer the decisions about a child to the parents. But the state must ensure that it "carries out its duty to protect its citizens but does not infringe on the rights granted to individuals by the First Amendment to the Constitution" (Black, 2006, para. 2). The state has a "high burden of proof" (para. 3) required before a parent loses guardianship of their child due to refusing medical treatment for a child. "If the proposed medical treatment has a good chance of success and the predicted outcome without treatment is death [and in some states suffering], courts are more likely to intervene and overrule parental decisions" (Black, 2006, para. 3). The concerned physicians must contact local state court systems (local judges) and request guardianship take place to provide lifesaving and essential medical treatments. The process of securing state guardianship can be rapid if the child's condition is deteriorating.

Guardians are responsible for (California Courts, 2020):

- Food, clothing, and shelter
- Safety and protection
- Physical and emotional growth
- Medical and dental care
- Education and special needs

Parents may have:

- A serious physical or mental illness
- The need to serve in the military or go overseas
- Gone to jail for a period of time
- A drug or alcohol problem
- A history of being abusive
- A lack of ability to care for their child for some reason

D LOSS OF PARENTAL GUARDIANSHIP

Here is a typical case example when courts secure guardianship for medical treatment decision and implementation against parental wishes (JUSTIA.US LAW, 2021). In the Court of Civil Appeals of Oklahoma (2001), the outcome for a young girl was favorable for the state to secure safety and treatment for a child. In the matter of D.R., the child suffered from seizure activity and developmental difficulties. While in physical therapy to address these problems, she experienced a severe seizure, after which her parents discontinued therapy and sought no other treatment. The state intervened, alleging medical neglect by the parent because the child's condition was potentially life-threatening.

This was a complicated case example when courts sided with Christian Scientist parents (Black, 2006):

> The Supreme Court of Delaware in *Newmark v. Williams* landed on the side of the parents. The child in *Newmark* was diagnosed with Burkitt's lymphoma and was given a 40% chance of survival if he obtained chemotherapy treatments. His parents decided that, rather than allowing an uncertain and painful medical treatment, they would seek treatment through their church. The state objected and filed for temporary custody (guardianship) of the child. The court determined that the parents were within their right to forgo the treatment. (para. 4)

> The spiritual treatment exemptions reflect, in part, 'the policy of this State with respect to the quality of life' a desperately ill child might have in the caring and loving atmosphere of his or her family, versus the sterile hospital environment demanded by physicians seeking to prescribe excruciating, and life-threatening, treatments of doubtful efficacy. (para. 6)

FIVE REASONS FOR COURTS TO OVERRIDE A PATIENT'S RIGHT TO REFUSE MEDICAL TREATMENT

Found in several US laws as reasons for courts to intervene and order treatments (Torrey, 2020; Vermontethicsnetwork.org, 2021):

1. Preservation of the life when the patient's condition is curable
2. Protection of the patient's dependents, especially minor children
3. Prevention of irrational self-destruction
4. Preservation of ethical integrity of healthcare providers
5. Protection of the public health and other interests

According to Diekema (2004), questions concerning conditions for justified state interference with parental decision-making have been identified as:

- By refusing to consent, are the parents placing their child at significant risk of serious harm?
- Is the harm imminent, requiring immediate action to prevent it?
- Is the intervention that has been refused necessary to prevent the serious harm?
- Is the intervention that has been refused of proven efficacy and therefore likely to prevent the harm?
- Does the intervention that has been refused by the parents not also place the child at significant risk of serious harm, and do its projected benefits outweigh its projected burdens significantly more favorably than the option chosen by the parents?

D LOSS OF PARENTAL GUARDIANSHIP

- Would any other option prevent serious harm to the child in a way that is less intrusive to parental autonomy and more acceptable to the parents?
- Can the state intervention be generalized to all other similar situations? Would most parents agree that the state intervention was reasonable?

APPENDIX E

COMMON CONCERNS ABOUT VACCINE ADMINISTRATION

Vaccine concerns, hesitancy, and refusal can range from 38 to 77% of parents (Linnard-Palmer, 2006; McKee & Bohannon, 2016). Healthcare professionals must be prepared to provide education. The following list includes concerns that parents may express to a healthcare provider. It is important to be prepared with an answer that is accurate and resources that are reputable:

- Fear of needle sticks, pain, and that my child will remember the experience and be traumatized.
- Vaccines will harm my child's immune system.
- Vaccines wear out an immune system.
- Vaccines are not properly tested for safety.
- Vaccines may cause side effects.
- Vaccines can cause iatrogenic effects (unwanted and untoward).

- Vaccines cause fevers.
- Vaccines cause allergic reactions, asthma, and even death.
- Vaccines cause developmental delays and/or learning disabilities.
- Vaccines, such as pertussis, cause brain damage.
- Vaccines may cause SIDS (sudden infant death syndrome).
- Vaccines are against my religion.
- Vaccines are against my culture.
- I have philosophical perspectives against childhood vaccines.
- I am concerned that the creation of the MMR vaccine uses aborted human fetal tissue.
- I am vegan, and vaccines use animal-derived gelatins.
- Worry of too many vaccines being given "too soon" or "too young."
- Worry that it is better to just give one immunization (shot) at a time per visit.
- Babies are already exposed to antigens, so why give more shots?
- Development of autism.
- My child will not be exposed to sexually transmitted infections, so why give HPV?
- Thimerosal is toxic or poisonous.
- Some vaccines cause type 1 diabetes.
- Vaccines can cause diseases like Crohn's, colitis, inflammatory bowel disease, and multiple sclerosis.
- Live vaccines can cause the very disease you are trying to prevent.

E COMMON CONCERNS ABOUT VACCINE ADMINISTRATION

- I can mitigate side effects by delaying my child's immunizations.
- Natural immunity is better, as we should not put foreign substances like vaccines in a child's body.
- Homeopathic solutions (aka nosodes) are a better alternative.
- My child doesn't need vaccines because no one gets these diseases anymore.
- My child doesn't need vaccines because those immunized children around us protect my child.
- My baby doesn't need vaccines because I am breastfeeding and will continue for months or years.

APPENDIX F

PANDEMICS AND TRUST IN RAPID VACCINE CREATION, DISTRIBUTION, AND MANDATES

The experience of a pandemic and the subsequent development of a vaccine can produce concerns for those who feel the vaccine development is "rushed" or "without sufficient safety in mind." Unfortunately, false advice on how and why to refuse vaccines circulated widely during pandemics such as smallpox (1905 mandate), NIHI influenza (mandated for healthcare professionals in 2009), SARS, and now COVID-19 (AFP Canada, 2020). During pandemics, some who are opposed to vaccines will state that the physician's Hippocratic Oath, or their code of professional ethics that pledges to cause no harm, is a basis of being able to "legally and ethically" refuse the administration of mandatory vaccines (AFP Canada, 2020). One source promotes the use of the claim that "all vaccines," include MRC-5, which they describe as aborted fetal cells and other DNA, is a basis for refusing mandatory vaccines for children and adults. According to the National Public Health Information Coalition, "Anti-vaxxers are terrified the government will 'enforce' a vaccine for coronavirus" (NPHIC, 2020, p. 1). Current literature states that around 50% of Americans plan on accepting a COVID-19 vaccine. This low vaccine expectancy will continue to allow the spread of the virus across the nation and the world.

The US has the strictest immunization policy examined, with legislation in all 50 states requiring vaccination for students and permanent residency applications (AFP Canada, 2020). As of the publication of this book, according to the National Conference of State Legislatures, 45 states and the District of Columbia grant exemptions on religious doctrine, 15 states have philosophical exemptions for moral, personal, or "other" beliefs (AFP Canada, 2020), and some employers allow for their healthcare providers to refuse annual influenza vaccines provided they wear a mask at all times at work from the beginning to the end of influenza season.

For further reading, see "False Advice on Refusing Vaccines Circulated During COVID-19 Pandemic" (AFP Canada, 2020, https://factcheck.afp.com/false-advice-refusing-vaccines-circulates-during-covid-19-pandemic) and "Is Mandatory Vaccination Legal in Time of Epidemic?" (Fujiwara, 2020, https://journalofethics.ama-assn.org/article/mandatory-vaccination-legal-time-epidemic/2006-04).

APPENDIX G

BEST INTEREST AND THE LAW: SHOULD STATE STATUTES ON CHILD ABUSE BE MODIFIED?

According to Hirasawa (2006), the complexity of the questions surrounding parental refusal of medical care for children for the application of beliefs requires a thoughtful evaluation of balancing individual freedom with the interference of government to potentially save a child's life and uphold the right of the child to be cared for. Hirasawa describes how there are varying degrees of the application of religion to medical treatment decisions and believes that parents "who make medical decisions based on religious beliefs should be liable for their child's death or disability if the use of conventional medicine and potential for recovery outweigh the probability that nonmedical treatment will cure the illness" (p. 1).

Should states that have exemptions statues on child abuse allowing the application of religion over traditional care be reviewed and modified to protect the child from harm, disability, and death? Whose best interest is at stake?

> Courts unanimously characterize the state's interest in protecting children as paramount, which justified burdening the parents' religious liberty. Therefore, parents should not be able to invoke a free exercise defense for failure to provide medical treatment for their children for serious medical conditions that are life-threatening or pose a substantial risk of harm to the child. (Hirasawa, 2006, p. 1)

APPENDIX H

SPIRITUAL ABUSE DEFINED

It is important to note that there is a reality to spiritual abuse. Again, not all of the 42 churches described in this book adhere to doctrines of such magnitude that one can consider the teachings dangerous and the followers abused, but there are cults that exist whose power over the followers can be interpreted as abusive. The delay or complete refusal of seeking medical care and treatment for children by church parishioners who are following coercive doctrine is an example of how influential some cults' teachings can be.

Circumstances of failure of parents to provide medical care and treatment to children have been known to cause severe disabilities, severe pain, and even death (AAP.org, 2013). The three top concerns surrounding the conflict of medicine and religion are summarized in the AAP policy statement and include: 1) religious exemptions to child neglect and abuse laws; 2) parental refusal of medical care and treatment for children; and 3) public funding for what is considered unproven spiritual and/or religious "healing practices" (AAP.org, 2013). To prevent a conflict that some consider spiritual abuse, or the application of religious doctrine taught by a religious or spiritual organization that conflicts with medical treatment leading to harm, professionals need to respect families' beliefs, collaborate with them, develop treatment plans, and work with child protective services as needed. Abuse caused by spiritual or religious organizations' doctrines must be addressed, including repealing religious exemptions to child neglect and child abuse laws (AAP.org, 2013).

APPENDIX I

RESOURCES FOR MORE INFORMATION

GENERAL RESOURCES

- Watch Tower Society publications for Jehovah's Witnesses
- Christian Science reading rooms
- Islamic Medical Association of North America (https://imana.org/)
- Book *Born in Zion* by former RN Carol Balizet, who promotes Christian home births, stating that medical care is linked to pagan witchcraft
- Advocates for Jehovah's Witness Reform on Blood (www.ajwrb.org)
- Elena Kondos's article "The Law and Christian Science Healing for Children: A Pathfinder" (1991) in *Legal Reference Services Quarterly*, 12(1), 5–71, gives detailed descriptions of exemptions, laws, beliefs, and resources for further study

- Rita Swan's article "Children, Medicine, Religion and the Law" (1997) in *Advances in Pediatrics*, 44, 491–544
- Book by yours truly, *When Parents Say No: Religious and Cultural Influences on Pediatric Healthcare Treatment* (2010), Sigma Theta Tau International Honor Society of Nursing

WEBSITES ON TREATMENT REFUSAL

- Children's Health Care is a Legal Duty (CHILD) (www.childrenshealthcare.org)
- Children's Health Care is a Legal Duty USA (www.CHILD.us.org)

USEFUL RESOURCES TO ASSIST IN THE MANAGEMENT OF PATIENTS WHO REFUSE BLOOD TRANSFUSIONS

- London Regional Transfusion Committee – Care Pathways for the Management of Adult Patients Refusing Blood (including Jehovah's Witnesses patients): https://www.transfusionguidelines.org/document-library/documents/care-pathways-for-the-management-of-adult-patients-refusing-blood-including-jehovah-s-witness-patients
- Better Blood Transfusion Toolkit – Pre-op Assessment for Jehovah's Witnesses: http://www.transfusionguidelines.org.uk/index.aspx?Publication=BBT&Section=22&pageid=1352

I RESOURCES FOR MORE INFORMATION

- The Royal College of Surgeons of England – Code of Practice for the Surgical Management of Jehovah's Witnesses: https://www.rcseng.ac.uk/library-and-publications/rcs-publications/docs/code-of-practice-for-the-surgical-management-of-jehovahs-witnesses/
- Developing a Blood Conservation Care Plan for Jehovah's Witness Patients with Malignant Disease: https://www.transfusionguidelines.org/document-library/documents/developing-a-blood-conservation-care-plan-for-jehovah-s-witness-patients-with-malignant-disease

RESOURCES AVAILABLE FOR CHILDREN, PARENTS, AND ADULTS REGARDING VACCINES

WEBSITES

American Academy of Pediatrics (AAP): www.aap.org/immunization

Centers for Disease Control and Prevention (CDC) for parents: www.cdc.gov/vaccines/parents; for healthcare providers: www.cdc.gov/vaccines

History of vaccines: www.historyofvaccines.org

Immunization Action Coalition (IAC) for the public: www.vaccineinformation.org; for healthcare providers: www.immunize.org

US Department of Health and Human Services (HHS): www.vaccines.gov

Vaccinate Your Family (formerly Every Child by Two): www.vaccinateyourfamily.org

Vaccine Education Center (VEC), Children's Hospital of Philadelphia: www.chop.edu/centers-programs/vaccine-education-center

Vaxopedia: www.vaxopedia.org/about/

Voices for Vaccines (VFV) for parents, other adults, and healthcare providers: www.voicesforvaccines.org

APPS FOR MOBILE DEVICES

Child Health Tracker: Developed by the American Academy of Pediatrics, this "tracker" gives parents the power of on-demand access to guidance on vaccinations and milestones they should be expecting with each birthday. Also included are tools like parent handouts for each well child visit. Available at a nominal cost from the AAP.

TravWell: Use this free app from the CDC to build a trip to get destination-specific vaccine recommendations, a checklist of what is needed to prepare for travel, and much more.

Vaccines on the Go—What You Should Know: This free app from the Vaccine Education Center at the Children's Hospital of Philadelphia provides parents with reliable information about the science, safety, and importance of vaccines and the diseases they prevent.

BOOKS FOR PARENTS

Baby 411, by Denise Fields and Ari Brown, Windsor Peak Press, 7th edition, 2015. Available from your favorite local or online bookstore.

I RESOURCES FOR MORE INFORMATION

Mama Doc Medicine: Finding Calm and Confidence in Parenting, Child Health, and World-Life Balance, by Wendy Sue Swanson, MD (aka "Seattle Mama Doc"), 2014. Available from the American Academy of Pediatrics at http://shop.aap.org/for-parents.

Parents Guide to Childhood Immunization, from the Centers for Disease Control and Prevention. Available at www.cdc.gov/vaccines/parents/tools/parents-guide/index.html to download or order.

Vaccine-Preventable Diseases: The Forgotten Story, by Texas Children's Hospital vaccine experts R. Cunningham et al. Available at www.tchorderprocessing.com to order.

Vaccines and Your Child, Separating Fact from Fiction, by Paul Offit, MD, and Charlotte Moser, Columbia University Press, 2011. Available at your favorite local or online bookstore.

VIDEOS

IAC's Video Library: Go to the Immunization Action Coalition's website for parents and the public, www.vaccineinformation.org/videos, for hundreds of video clips about vaccines and vaccine preventable diseases.

Shot by Shot Video Collection: Go to www.shotbyshot.org to read people's stories of vaccine-preventable diseases shared on the California Immunization Coalition website.

PHONE NUMBERS

CDC-INFO Contact Center: Operated by the Centers for Disease Control and Prevention, this number is for both members of the general public and healthcare professionals who have questions about immunization and vaccine preventable diseases. Call (800) CDC-INFO or (800) 232-4636. TTY: (888) 232-6348. CDC-INFO's operating hours are Monday through Friday from 8 a.m. to 8 p.m. (ET).

REFERENCES

AAP.org. (2018). *Immunizations: Common parental concerns*. https://www.aap.org/en-us/advocacy-and-policy/aap-health-initiatives/immunizations/Pages/Common-Parental-Concerns.aspx

Adams, C. E., & Leverland, M. B. (1986). The effects of religious beliefs on the health care practices of the Amish. *Nurse Practitioner, 11*(3), 58, 63, 67. doi:10.1097.00006205-198603000-00008

Advocates for Jehovah's Witnesses for Reform on Blood. (1998). *The president of the Constitutional Court of Colombia affirms that denying a blood transfusion constitutes first degree murder*. http://watchtower-blood.org/newsmedia/sd/sd_eng.shtml

Advocates for Jehovah's Witnesses for Reform on Blood. (2017). *Blood transfusion – is it a meal?* www.ajwrb.org/is-a-blood-transfusion-a-meal

Advocates for Jehovah's Witnesses for Reform on Blood. (2020). *Do Jehovah's Witnesses really abstain from blood?* https://www.ajwrb.org/do-jehovahs-witnesses-really-abstain-from-blood

AFP Canada. (2020). *False advice on refusing vaccines circulated during COID-19 pandemic*. https://factcheck.afp.com/false-advice-refusing-vaccines-circulates-during-covid-19-pandemic

Ahmedani, B. K., Peterson, E. L., Wells, K. E., Rand, C. S., & Williams, L. K. (2013). Asthma medication adherence: The role of God and other health locus of control factors. *Annals of Allergy, Asthma, & Immunology, 110*, 75–79. http://dx.doi.org/10.1016/j.anai.2012.11.006

Akoum, M. E. (2019). *4 reasons why parents are refusing to vaccinate their children, and 4 reasons why they (really) shouldn't*. https://www.wish.org.qa/blog/4-reasons-why-parents-are-refusing-to-vaccinate-their-children-and-4-reasons-why-they-really-shouldnt/

Alfandre, D. (2013). Reconsidering against medical advice discharges: Embracing patient-centeredness to promote high quality care and a renewed research agenda. *Journal of General Internal Medicine, 28*(12), 1657–1662.

Alfandre, D., & Schumann, J. (2013). What is wrong with discharges against medical advice (and how to fix them). *JAMA, 310*(22), 2393–2394. doi:10.1001/jama.2013.280887

American Academy of Pediatrics. (2013). Policy statement: Conflicts between religious or spiritual beliefs and pediatric care: Informed refusal, exemptions and public funding. *Pediatrics, 132*(5), 962–955. doi:10.1542/peds.2013-2716

American Academy of Pediatrics Committee on Bioethics. (1995). Informed consent, parental permission, and assent in pediatric practice. *Pediatrics, 95*(2), 314–317.

American Academy of Pediatrics Committee on Bioethics. (1997). Religious objections of medical care. *Pediatrics, 99*(2), 279–281.

American Academy of Pediatrics Committee on Bioethics. (2013). Conflicts between religious or spiritual beliefs and pediatric care: Informed refusal, exemptions, and public funding. *Pediatrics, 132*(5), 962–965. https://doi.org/10.1542/peds.2013-2716

American Academy of Pediatrics Committee on Bioethics. (2016). Informed consent in decision making in pediatric practice. *Pediatrics, 138*(2), e20161484.

American Heart Association News. (2019). *Health disparities—even in the face of socioeconomic success—baffle experts.* https://www.heart.org/en/news/2019/02/13/health-disparities-even-in-the-face-of-socioeconomic-success-baffle-experts

American Medical Association. (2019). *AMA policy advocates to eliminate non-medical vaccine exemptions.* https://www.ama-assn.org/press-center/press-releases/ama-policy-advocates-eliminate-non-medical-vaccine-exemptions

Anderson, G. R. (1983). Medicine vs. religion: The case of Jehovah's Witnesses. *Health and Social Work, 8*, 31–38.

Appelbaum, P., & Roth, L. (1983). Patients who refuse treatment in medical hospitals. *JAMA, 250*(10), 1296–1301.

Asser, S. M., & Swan, R. (1998). Child fatalities from religion-motivated medical neglect. *Pediatrics, 101*(4), 625–629. https://doi.org/10.1542/peds.101.4.625

Avent, J. R., Cashwell, C. S., & Brown-Jeffy, S. (2015). African American pastors on mental health, coping, and help seeking. *Counseling and Values, 60,* 32–47. https://doi.org/10.1002/j.2161-007X.2015.00059.x

Baker Eddy, M. (1875). *Science and health* [reprint of historic 1st edition]. Create Space Publishing.

Barnes, P., Powell-Griner, E., McFann, K., & Nahin, R. (2004). Complementary and alternative medicine use among adults: United States, 2002. *Advance Data From Vital and Health Statistics, 343,* 1–19.

Belz, E. (2019). *When the fog lifts.* World News Group. https://wng.org/articles/when-the-fog-lifts-1620590821

Black, L. (2006). Limiting parents' rights in medical decision making. *AMA Journal of Ethics, 8*(10), 676–680. doi:10.1001/virtualmentor.2006.8.10.hlaw1-0610

Blewett, L., Rivera Drew, J., Griffin, R., King, M., & Williams, K. (2016). *IPUMS health surveys: National Health Interview Survey, Version 6.2.* Minneapolis, MN: University of Minnesota. https://www.ipums.org/projects/ipums-health-surveys/d070.v6.2

Brenan, M. (2018, December 24). *Religion considered important to 72% of Americans.* Gallup Poll. https://news.gallup.com/poll/245651/religion-considered-important-americans.aspx

REFERENCES

Brown, R. (2020, February 17). Faith healing and Idaho law. *The Idaho Statesman.*

Brown University. (2021). *Philosophy: What and why?* https://www.brown.edu/academics/philosophy/undergraduate/philosophy-what-and-why

California Courts. (2020). *Guardianship.* https://www.courts.ca.gov/selfhelp-guardianship.htm

Canadian Paediatric Society. (2004). Treatment decisions regarding infants, children and adolescents. *Paediatrics & Child Health, 9*(2), 99–114. https://doi.org/10.1093/pch/9.2.99

Caringforkids.cps.ca. (2016). *Vaccines: Common concerns.* https://www.caringforkids.cps.ca/handouts/vaccines-common-concerns

Catlin, A. (1997). Commentary of Johnny's story: Transfusing a Jehovah's Witness. *Pediatric Nursing, 23*(3), 289–291, 317.

Centers for Disease Control and Prevention. (2010). Prenatal and infant exposure to thimerosal from vaccines and immunoglobins and risk of autism. *Pediatrics, 126*(4), 656–664. doi: 10.1542/peds.2010-0309

Centers for Disease Control and Prevention. (2016a). *For immunization managers: State vaccination requirements.* https://www.cdc.gov/vaccines/imz-managers/laws/state-reqs.html

Centers for Disease Control and Prevention. (2016b). *History of small pox.* https://www.cdc.gov/smallpox/history/history.html

Centers for Disease Control and Prevention. (2018). *Vaccination laws.* https://www.cdc.gov/phlp/publications/topic/vaccinationlaws.html

Centers for Disease Control and Prevention. (2019a). *Conjunctivitis (pink eye) in newborns.* https://www.cdc.gov/conjunctivitis/newborns.html

Centers for Disease Control and Prevention. (2019b). *Racial and ethnic disparities continue in pregnancy-related deaths* [News release]. https://www.cdc.gov/media/releases/2019/p0905-racial-ethnic-disparities-pregnancy-deaths.html

Centers for Disease Control and Prevention. (2019c). *Talking points on health literacy.* https://www.cdc.gov/healthliteracy/shareinteract/TellOthers.html

Centers for Disease Control and Prevention. (2020a). *Guillain-Barré Syndrome and vaccines.* www.cdc.gov/vaccinesafety/concerns/guillain-barre-syndrome.html

Centers for Disease Control and Prevention. (2020b). *Measles history.* https://www.cdc.gov/measles/about/history.html

Centers for Disease Control and Prevention. (2020c). *Vaccine safety: Thimerosal and vaccines.* https://www.cdc.gov/vaccinesafety/concerns/thimerosal/index.html

Centers for Disease Control and Prevention. (2021a). *Covid data tracker.* https://covid.cdc.gov/covid-data-tracker/#vaccinations_vacc-total-admin-rate-total

Centers for Disease Control and Prevention. (2021b). *Measles (rubeola) cases and outbreaks.* https://www.cdc.gov/measles/cases-outbreaks.html

Centers for Disease Control and Prevention. (2021c). *Understanding mRNA vaccines.* https://www.cdc.gov/coronavirus/2019-ncov/vaccines/different-vaccines/mRNA.html?s_cid=10506:how%20does%20mrna%20vaccine%20work:sem.ga:p:RG:GM:gen:PTN:FY21

Chand, N. K., Subramanya, H. B., & Rao, G. V. (2014). Management of patients who refuse blood transfusion. *Indian Journal of Anesthesia, 58*(5), 658–664.

CHILD USA. (n.d.). *Religious exemptions to medical treatment of children in state civil & criminal codes.* http://childrenshealthcare.org/?page_id=24

CHILD USA. (2020). *Neglect and maltreatment.* https://childusa.org/medicalneglect/

CHILD USA. (2021). *Ethics of testing and screening requirements.* childusa.org/wp-content/uploads/2020/03/screeningethics.pdf

Children's Hospital of Philadelphia. (2020). *Vaccine ingredients – fetal cells.* https://www.chop.edu/centers-programs/vaccine-education-center/vaccine-ingredients/fetal-tissues

Choi, M., Kim, H., Qian, H., & Palepu, A. (2011). Readmission rates of patients discharged against medical advice: A matched cohort study. *PLOS One,* 6e24459. https://doi.org/10.1371/journal.pone.0024459

Chojnowski, K., Janus, A., Bli niewska, K., Robak, M., & Treli ski, J. (2016). Long lasting extreme anemia during the therapy of acute lymphoblastic leukemia in a Jehovah's Witness patient. *Transfusion, 56*(10), 2438–2442. doi: 10.1111/trf.13703

Christianscience.com. (2020). *Insurance and Christian Science.* https://www.christianscience.com/additional-resources/committee-on-publication/u.s.-federal-office/insurance-and-christian-science

Christianscience.com. (2021a). *What is Christian Science?* Mary Baker Eddy. https://www.christianscience.com/what-is-christian-science/mary-baker-eddy

Christianscience.com. (2021b). *Christian Science nursing: The ministry of Christian Science nursing.* www.christianscience.com/additional-resources/christian-science-nursing

Clutter, L. (2005). Spiritual issues in children's health-care settings. In J. A. Rollins, R. Bolig., & C. C. Mahan (Eds.), *Meeting children's psychosocial needs across the health-care continuum* (pp. 351–420). Pro-ED, Inc.

Cohen, M., Shaykevich, S., Cawthon, C., Kripalani, S., Paasche-Orlow, M., & Schnipper, J. (2012). Predictors of medication adherence postdischarge: The impact of patient age, insurance status, and prior adherence. *Journal of Hospital Medicine.* https://onlinelibrary.wiley.com/doi/abs/10.1002/jhm.1940

College of Physicians of Philadelphia. (2021). *The history of vaccines: Cultural perspectives on vaccination.* https://www.historyofvaccines.org/content/articles/cultural-perspectives-vaccination

Corley, M., Elswick, R., & Gorman, M. (2001). Development and evaluation of a moral distress scale. *Journal of Advanced Nursing, 33*(2), 250–256.

REFERENCES

Cornell Law School. (2020). *The belief-conduct distinction.* https://www.law.cornell.edu/constitution-conan/amendment-1/the-belief-conduct-distinction

Crombie, N. (2019, Jan. 9). Followers of Christ criminal investigations: A history. *The Oregonian/Oregon Live.* https://www.oregonlive.com/oregon-city/2017/03/followers_of_christ_investigat.html

Cruzan by Cruzan v. Director, Missouri Department of Health. (1989). https://www.oyez.org/cases/1989/88-1503

Cult Education Institute. (2014). *Followers of Christ.* https://culteducation.com/group/925-followers-of-christ.html

Curlin, F., Roach, C., Gorawara-Bhat, R., Lantos, J., & Chin, M. (2005). When patients choose faith over medicine: Physician perspectives on religiously related conflict in the medical encounter. *Archives of Internal Medicine, 165*(1), 88–91. doi:10.1001/archinte.165.1.88

Cushing, M. (1982). Whose best interest? Parents vs. child rights. *American Journal of Nursing, 82*(2), 313–315.

Davidson, E., Lam, S., & Sokn, E. (2019). Predictors of medication nonadherence from outpatient pharmacy data within a large, academic health system. *Journal of Pharmacy Practice, 32*(2), 175–178.

Davis, M., & Fang, A. (2020). *Emancipated minor.* StatPearls Publishing. https://www.ncbi.nlm.nih.gov/books/NBK554594/

Deer, B. (2011). Secrets of the MMR scare. How the vaccine crisis was meant to make money. *British Medical Journal, 342,* c5258.

DeJesus, I. (2017). *God's will vs. medicine: Does Faith Tabernacle beliefs put children at risk?* https://www.pennlive.com/news/2017/02/faith_healing_faith_tabernacle.html

Del Buono, A. (2016). Living on a prayer: Faith healers escaping criminal liability for child abuse through religious affirmative defenses & exemption laws. *Rutgers Journal of Law & Religion, 17,* 452–453. https://www.lawandreligion.com/sites/law-religion/files/Living-On-A-Prayer-Del-Buono.pdf

Denzin, J., & Lincoln, Y. (2000). *Handbook of qualitative research* (2nd ed.). Sage Publications.

Diekema, D. S. (2004). Parental refusals of medical treatment: The harm principle as threshold for state intervention. *Theoretical Medicine, 25,* 243–264.

Dodes, I. (1987). Suffer the little children . . . toward a judicial recognition of duty of reasonable care owed children by religious faith healers. *Hofstra Law Review, 16,* 165–190.

Dusek, J., Astin, J., Hibberd, P., & Krucoff, M. (2003). Healing prayer outcomes studies: Consensus recommendations. *Alternative Therapies, 9*(3), A44–A53.

Dwyer, J. (1996). The children we abandon: Religious exemptions to child welfare and education laws as denials of equal protection to children of religious objectors. *North Carolina Law Review, 74,* 1321–1478.

Dyer, J. (2000). Affordable housing vs. mass transit. *Boulder Weekly.* www.boulderweekly.com/archive/030101/dyertimes

Edberg, M. (2013). *Essentials of health behavior: Social and behavioral theory in public health* (6th ed.). Jones & Bartlett.

Eddy, M. B. (1875). *Science and health with key to the scriptures.* The Christian Science Publishing Society.

Eggertson, L. (2010). Lancet retracts 12-year-old article linking autism to MMR vaccines. *Canadian Medical Association Journal, 182*(4), E199–E200. https://doi.org/10.1503/cmaj.109-3179

Farson, K., & Cunnynham, K. (2016). *Trends in supplemental nutrition assistance program participation rates: Fiscal year 2010 to fiscal year 2014.* Washington, DC: US Department of Agriculture, Food and Nutrition Service. https://fns-prod.azureedge.net/sites/default/files/ops/Trends2010-2014.pdf

Fink, A. S., Prochazka, A. V, Henderson, W. G., Bartenfeld, D., Nyirenda, C., Webb, A., . . . Parmelee, P. (2010). Predictors of comprehension during surgical informed consent. *Journal of the American College of Surgeons, 210*(6), 919–926.

Flannery, E. (1995). One advocate's viewpoint. *Journal of Law Medicine and Ethics, 23*(1), 7–12.

Foreman, D. M. (1999). The family rule: Framework for obtaining ethical consent. *Journal of Medical Ethics, 25*(6), 491–496.

Fost, N. (1981). Ethical issues in the treatment of critically ill newborns. *Pediatric Annals, 10*(10), 16–52.

Fox, V. (1990). Caught between religion and medicine. *AORN, 52*(1), 131–146.

Foy, N., & Pfannenstiel, K. (2018). Coroner's primary reignites faith healing debate. *Idaho Press.* https://www.idahopress.com/news/local/2cscoop/coroners-primary-reignites-faith-healing-debate/article_50acec6d-21ba-57fd-935d-60c3b9c1a2a1.html

Fujiwara, S. (2020). Is mandatory vaccination legal in time of epidemic? *American Medical Association Journal of Ethics.* https://journalofethics.ama-assn.org/article/mandatory-vaccination-legal-time-epidemic/2006-04

Gabbatt, A. (2020). U.S. anti-vaxxers aim to spread fear over future coronavirus vaccine. *The Guardian.* https://www.theguardian.com/world/2020/may/29/anti-vaxxers-fight-against-coronavirus

Gamble, B. N. (1997). Under the shadow of Tuskegee: African Americans and health care. *American Journal of Public Health, 87*(11), 1773–1778.

Gill, D. (2021). *From the frontlines: Understanding herd immunity.* https://www.lung.org/blog/understanding-covid-herd-immunity

Gillon, R. (1994). Medical ethics: Four principles plus attention to scope. *British Medical Journal, 309*, 184. https://doi.org/10.1136/bmj.309.6948.184

REFERENCES

Gillum, R. F. (2013). From papyrus to the electronic tablet: A brief history of the clinical medical record with lessons for the digital age. *The American Journal of Medicine, 126*(10), 853–857. doi:10.1016/j.amjmed.2013.03.024

Giubilini, A., Douglas, T., & Savulescu, J. (2018). The moral obligation to be vaccinated: Utilitarianism, contractualism, and collective easy rescue. *Medicine, Health Care, and Philosophy, 21*(4), 547–560. https://doi.org/10.1007/s11019-018-9829-y

Glover, R. J., & Rushton, C. (1995). Introducing: From Baby Doe to Baby K. *Journal of Law, Medicine & Ethics, 23*, 5–6.

Godfrey, A. (2017). Leaving against medical advice (AMA): A clinician's dilemma. *NEJM Journal Watch.* https://blogs.jwatch.org/frontlines-clinical-medicine/2017/05/11/leaving-medical-advice-ama-clinicians-dilemma/

Godlee, F. (2011). The fraud behind the MMR scare. *British Medical Journal, 342*, d22.

Gorn, D. (2017). *Food as medicine: It's not just a fringe idea anymore.* https://www.npr.org/sections/thesalt/2017/01/17/509520895/food-as-medicine-it-s-not-just-a-fringeideaanymore#:~:text=The%20food%2Das%2Dmedicine%20movement,than%20relying%20solely%20on%20medications

Green, A. (2019, Aug. 29). Are decades of needless child deaths a thing of the past for the Followers of Christ? *The Oregonian/OregonLive.* https://www.oregonlive.com/news/erry-2018/07/c6430fe46a2145/are-decades-of-needless-child.html

Greenawalt, K. (2008). *The cultural defense: Reflections in light of the model penal code and the Religious Freedom Restoration Act.* https://kb.osu.edu/bitstream/handle/1811/73066/OSJCL_V6N1_299.pdf

Grimes, D. R. (2019). *Good thinking: Why flawed logic puts us all at risk and how critical thinking can save the world.* The Experiment LLC.

Grimes, D. R. (2020). *Combatting vaccine hesitancy and disinformation: Lessons from the case of HVP vaccine in Ireland* [Presentation to NVAC]. https://www.hhs.gov/sites/default/files/nvac_feb2020_day2_panel3-v1.pdf

Grootens-Wiegers, P., Hein, I. M., van den Broek, J. M., & de Vries, M. C. (2017). Medical decision-making in children and adolescents: Developmental and neuroscientific aspects. *BMC Pediatrics, 17*(1), 120. https://doi.org/10.1186/s12887-017-0869-x

Gündüz, R. C., Halil, H., Gürsoy, C., Çifci, A., Özgün, S., Kodaman, T., & Sönmez, M. (2014). Refusal of medical treatment in the pediatric emergency services: Analysis of reasons and aspects. *Turkish Journal of Pediatrics, 56*(6), 638–642.

Haines, K., Freeman, J., Vastaas, C., Rust, C., Cox, C., Kasotakis, G., . . . Agarwal, S. (2019). "I'm leaving": Factors that impact against medical advice disposition post-trauma. *Journal of Emergency Medicine, 58*(4), 691–697.

Hamel, L., Kirzinger, A., Lopes, L., Kearney, A., Sparks, G., & Brodie, M. (2021). Vaccine hesitancy. *KFF COVID-19 Vaccine Monitor.* https://www.kff.org/report-section/kff-covid-19-vaccine-monitor-january-2021-vaccine-hesitancy/

Hamilton, D. (2017). *Why, despite post-racial rhetoric, do racial health disparities increase at higher income levels?* Washington Center for Equitable Growth. https://equitablegrowth.org/post-racial-rhetoric-racial-health-disparities-and-health-disparity-consequences-of-stigma-stress-and-racism/

Hammersley, M., & Atkinson, P. (1993). *Ethnography: Principles in practice* (2nd ed.). Routledge.

Hanna, D. R. (2004). Moral distress: The state of the science. *Research and Theory for Nursing Practice, 18*(1), 73–93. doi: 10.1891/rtnp.18.1.73.28054

Harrison, C., Canadian Paediatric Society, & Bioethics Committee. (2004). Treatment decisions regarding infants, children and adolescents. *Paediatrics & Child Health, 9*(2), 99–103. https://doi.org/10.1093/pch/9.2.99

Heller, J. (2005, Sept. 13). Is it freedom vs. responsibility? *Tampa Bay Times.* https://www.tampabay.com/archive/1998/10/01/is-it-freedom-vs-responsibility/

Herrskink, O. (2020, January 18). *Panel calls for changes in Idaho's faith-healing exemptions during 2020 session.* KHOU-TV. https://www.khou.com/article/news/local/capitol-watch/panel-calls-for-changes-to-idahos-faith-healing-exemption-during-2020-session/277-75b4ec60-c6dd-472c-8a3d-f32175bddb59

HHS.gov. (2020). *Vaccines and Immunizations.* https://www.hhs.gov/vaccines/index.html

Hilts, P. J. (1998, April 15). Experiments on children are reviewed. *The New York Times.* https://www.nytimes.com/1998/04/15/nyregion/experiments-on-children-are-reviewed.html

Hirasawa, K. R. (2006). Are parents acting in the best interests for their children when they make medical decisions based on their religious beliefs? *Family Court Review, 44*(2), 316–329.

Hofstede, G. (1985). The interaction between national and organizational value systems [1]. *Journal of Management Studies, 22,* 347–357. https://doi.org/10.1111/j.1467-6486.1985.tb00001.x

Hooper, L., Huffman, L., Higginbotham, J., Mugoya, G., Smith, A., & Dumas, T. (2018). Associations among depressive symptoms, wellness, patient involvement, provider cultural competency, and treatment nonadherence: A pilot study among community patients seen at a university medical center. *Community Mental Health Journal, 54*(2), 138–148.

Hotz, K. G. (2015). "Big momma had sugar, imma have it too": Medical fatalism and the language of faith among African-American women in Memphis. *Journal of Religion and Health, 54,* 2212–2224. https://doi.org/10.1007/s10943-014-9969-1

Humber, J. M., & Almeder, R. F. (2000). *Is there a duty to die?* Humana Press.

Huntsberry-Lett, A. (2020). *Know your rights: Understanding hospital discharge against medical advice.* https://www.agingcare.com/articles/know-your-rights-understanding-hospital-discharges-against-medical-advice-445934.htm

REFERENCES

Ibeneme, S., Eni, G., Ezuma, A., & Fortwengel, G. (2017). Roads to health in developing countries: Understanding the intersection of culture and healing. *Current Therapeutic Research*, 86, 13–18. https://www.sciencedirect.com/science/article/pii/S0011393X17300036

Idahochildren.org. (2020). *Child abuse in Idaho: Deadly and legal.* http://idahochildren.org/

Immunization Action Coalition. (2019). *Reliable sources of immunization information: Where parents can go to find answers!* https://www.immunize.org/catg.d/p4012.pdf

Institute of Medicine (US) Committee on the Use of Complementary and Alternative Medicine by the American Public. (2005). *Complementary and alternative medicine in the United States.* Washington, DC: National Academies Press. https://www.ncbi.nlm.nih.gov/books/NBK83799/

Institute for Vaccine Safety (Johns Hopkins Bloomberg School of Public Health). (2018). *Do vaccines cause meningitis or encephalitis?* https://www.vaccinesafety.edu/vs-mening.htm

Jameton, A. (1993) Dilemmas of moral distress: Moral responsibility and nursing practice. *Clinical Issues in Perinatal and Women's Health Nursing*, 4, 542–551.

Janofsky, M. (2001, Feb. 21). Colorado children's deaths rekindle debate on religion. *The New York Times.* https://www.nytimes.com/2001/02/21/us/colorado-children-s-deaths-rekindle-debate-on-religion.html

Johns Hopkins Medicine. (2020). *Measles: What you should know.* https://www.hopkinsmedicine.org/health/conditions-and-diseases/measles-what-you-should-know

Joint United Kingdom (UK) Blood Transfusion and Tissue Transplantation Services Professional Advisory Committee. (2020a). *6: Alternatives and adjuncts to blood transfusion.* https://www.transfusionguidelines.org/transfusion-handbook/6-alternatives-and-adjuncts-to-blood-transfusion

Joint United Kingdom (UK) Blood Transfusion and Tissue Transplantation Services Professional Advisory Committee. (2020b). *12.2: Jehovah's Witnesses and blood transfusion.* https://www.transfusionguidelines.org/transfusion-handbook/12-management-of-patients-who-do-not-accept-transfusion/12-2-jehovah-s-witnesses-and-blood-transfusion

Juckett, G. (2005). Cross-cultural medicine. *American Family Physician*, 72(11), 2267–2274. https://www.aafp.org/afp/2005/1201/p2267.html

JUSTIA.US Law. (2021). IN RE: D. R. 2001 OK CIV APP 21. law.justia.com/cases/oklahoma/court-of-appeals-civil/2001/182908.html

JW.org. (2021). *How many of Jehovah's Witnesses are there worldwide?* https://www.jw.org/en/jehovahs-witnesses/faq/how-many-jw/

KFF COVID-19 Vaccine Monitor. (2021). *An ongoing research project tracking the public's attitudes and experiences with COVID-19 vaccinations.* https://www.kff.org/coronavirus-covid-19/dashboard/kff-covid-19-vaccine-monitor-dashboard/?utm_source=web&utm_medium=trending&utm_campaign=COVID-19-vaccine-monitor)

Koenig H. G. (2012). Religion, spirituality, and health: The research and clinical implications. *International Scholarly Research Notices, 2012*, 278730. https://doi.org/10.5402/2012/278730

Kondos, E. (1992) The law and Christian Science healing for children: A pathfinder. *Legal Reference Services Quarterly, 12*(1), 5–71.

Kopelman, L., Irons, T., & Kopelman, A. (1988). Neonatologists judge the "Baby Doe" regulations. *The New England Journal of Medicine, 318*(11), 677–683.

Kostinchuk, D. (2001). *Faith healing: Child abuse, torture and homicide.* https://infidels.org/kiosk/article/faith-healing-child-abuse-torture-and-homicide-104.html

Kraszewski, J., Burke, T., & Rosenbaum, S. (2006). Legal issues in newborn screening: Implications for public health practice and policy. *Public Health Reports, 121*(1), 92–94. https://doi.org/10.1177/003335490612100116

Kraut, A., Fransoo, R., Olafson, K., Ramsay, C., Yogendran, M., & Garland, A. (2013). A population-based analysis of leaving the hospital against medical advice: Incidence and associated variables. *BMC Health Services Research, 13*, 415. https://doi.org/10.1186/1472-6963-13-415

Lantos, J., & Miles, S. (1989) Autonomy in adolescent medicine: A framework for decisions about life-sustaining treatment. *Journal of Adolescent Healthcare, 10*(6), 460–468.

Larabee, M. (1998, Nov. 28). The battle over faith healing: When prayer pre-empts medical care, prosecutors nationwide struggle to respect parents' freedoms while protecting children's lives. *The Oregonian.* https://culteducation.com/group/925-followers-of-christ/7140-the-battle-over-faith-healing.html

Lawry, K., Slomka, J., & Goldfarb, J. (1996). What went wrong: Multiple perspectives on an adolescent's decision to refuse blood transfusions. *Clinical Pediatrics, 35*(6), 317–322.

LeCompte, M., & Schensul, J. (1999). *The ethnographer's tool kit.* AltaMira Press.

Lee, C., Cho, J., Choi, S., Kim, H., & Park J. (2016). Patients who leave the emergency department against medical advice. *Clinical and Experimental Emergency Medicine, 3*(2), 88–94.

Leininger, M., & McFarland, M. (2002). *Transcultural nursing: Concepts, theories, research and practice* (3rd ed.). McGraw-Hill.

Lerner, M. (1994). *Choices in healing: Integrating the best of conventional and complementary approaches to cancer.* MIT Press.

Levin, J. (1994). Religion and health: Is there an association, is it valid, and is it causal? *Social Science Medicine, 38*(11), 1475–1482.

Linnard-Palmer, L. (2006). *When parents say no: Religious and cultural influences on pediatric healthcare treatment.* Sigma Theta Tau International.

Linnard-Palmer, Luanne. (2021). *Refusal of medical treatment due to religious and cultural beliefs: Use of power distance to influence pediatric care outcomes* [Manuscript submitted for publication].

REFERENCES

Linnard-Palmer, L., & Coats, G. (2010). *Safe maternity and pediatric nursing.* FA Davis Publishing Company.

Linnard-Palmer, L., & Coats, G. (2021). *Safe maternity and pediatric nursing* (2nd ed.). FA Davis Publishing Company.

Linnard-Palmer, L., & Kools, S. (2004). Parents' refusal of medical treatment based on religious and/or cultural beliefs: The law, ethical principles, and clinical implications. *Journal of Pediatric Nursing, 19*(5), 351–356.

Linnard-Palmer, L., & Kools, S. (2005). Parents' refusal of medical treatment for cultural or religious beliefs: An ethnographic study of healthcare professionals' experiences. *Journal of Pediatric Oncology Nursing, Jan, 22,* 4–57.

Lipson, J., Dibble, S., & Minarik, P. (1996). *Culture and nursing care: A pocket guide.* UCSF Nursing Press.

Lloyd, J., Maresh, S., Powers, C., Shrank, W., & Alley, D. (2019). How much does medication nonadherence cost the Medicare fee-for-service program? *Medical Care, 57*(3), 218–224.

Loma Linda University Health. (n.d.-a). *Findings for lifestyle, diet & disease.* https://adventisthealthstudy.org/studies/AHS-2/findings-lifestyle-diet-disease

Loma Linda University Health. (n.d.-b). *Lifestyle medicine specialist fellowship.* https://lluh.org/health-professionals/gme/resident-fellow/lifestyle-medicine-specialist-fellowship

Loskutova, N., Smail, C., Callen, E., Staton, E., Nazir, N., Webster, B., & Pace, W. (2020). Effects of multicomponent primary care-based intervention on immunization rates and missed opportunities to vaccinate adults. *BMC Family Practice, 21,* 46. https://doi.org/10.1186/s12875-020-01115-y

Lu, D. W., & Adams, J. G. (2009). Ethical issues. In R. R. Bass (Ed.), *Medical oversight of EMS* (pp. 117–124). Kendall/Hunt Publishing Company.

Lybarger v. People. (1991). Supreme Court of Colorado, 807, P.2d 570. https://casetext.com/case/lybarger-v-people

Macklin, R. (1988). The inner workings of an ethics committee: Latest battle over Jehovah's Witnesses. *Hasting Center Report, 18*(1), 15–20.

Mann, M., Votto, J., Kambe, J., & McNamee, M. (1992). Management of the severely anemic patient who refuses transfusion: Lessons learned during the care of a Jehovah's Witness. *Annals of Internal Medicine, 117*(2), 1043–1048.

Massachusetts Citizens for Children. (2021). *Exemption laws lead to the cruel and unnecessary deaths of helpless children: These laws also falsely mislead parents regarding their legal duty to provide necessary medical care for their seriously ill children.* https://www.masskids.org/index.php/religious-exemption-laws-lead-to-cruel-deaths-mislead-parents

Mayoclinic.org. (2019). *Lead poisoning: Overview.* www.mayoclinic.org/diseases-conditions/lead-poisoning/symptoms-causes/syc-20354717

McKee, C., & Bohannon, K. (2016). Exploring the reasons behind parental refusal of vaccines. *The Journal of Pediatric Pharmacology and Therapeutics, 21*(2), 104–109. https://doi.org/10.5863/1551-6776-21.2.104

Melton, J. G. (2014, June 26). *Jehovah's Witness.* https://www.britannica.com/topic/Jehovahs-Witnesses

Menendez, M., van Dijk, C., & Ring, D. (2015). Who leaves the hospital against medical advice in the orthopaedic setting? *Clinical Orthopaedics and Related Research, 473,* 1140–1149. https://link.springer.com/article/10.1007%2Fs11999-014-3924-z

Migden, D., & Braen, G. (1998). The Jehovah's Witness blood refusal care: Ethical and medicolegal considerations for emergency physicians. *Academic Emergency Medicine, 5,* 815–824.

Miller, W. R., & Rollnick, S. (2013). *Motivational interviewing: Helping people change* (3rd ed.). Guilford Press.

MindTools.com. (n.d.). *Hofstede's cultural dimensions: Understanding different countries.* https://www.mindtools.com/pages/article/newLDR_66.htm

Monopoli, P. (1991). Allocating the costs of parental free exercise: Striking a balance between sincere religious belief and a child's right to medical treatment. *Pepperdine Law Review, 18,* 319–352.

Monroe, K., Skocyzylas, M. S., & Burrows, H. L. (2018). When parents say "no" to newborn nursery protocols. *Contemporary Pediatrics.* https://www.contemporarypediatrics.com/view/when-parents-say-no-newborn-nursery-protocols

Morning Consult Poll. (2020). *The U.S. is struggling to contain coronavirus. Voters have taken notice.* https://morningconsult.com/2020/03/02/coronavirus-trump-approval-decline-poll/

Munoz, D., Llamas, L., & Bosch-Capblanch, X. (2015). Exposing concerns about vaccination in low- and middle-income countries: A systematic review. *International Journal of Public Health, 60*(7), 767–780. doi: 10.1007/s00038-015-0715-6

Muramoto, O. (1999). Recent developments in medical care of Jehovah's Witnesses. *World Journal of Medicine, 5*(170), 297–301.

National Cancer Institute. (2020). *Children's assent.* https://www.cancer.gov/about-cancer/treatment/clinical-trials/patient-safety/childrens-assent

National Conference of State Legislatures. (2020). *States with religious and philosophical exemptions from school immunization requirements.* https://www.ncsl.org/research/health/school-immunization-exemption-state-laws.aspx

National Health Service. (2017). *Do I have the right to refuse treatment?* https://www.nhs.uk/common-health-questions/nhs-services-and-treatments/do-i-have-the-right-to-refuse-treatment/

National Public Health Information Coalition. (2020). *Anti-vax groups fear a coronavirus vaccine.* https://www.nphic.org/nphichighlights/3918-newshighlight-8

REFERENCES

Natural Resources Defense Council. (2019). *Flint water crisis: Everything you need to know.* www.nrdc.org/stories/flint-water-crisis-everything-you-need-know#sec-summary

Neely, G. (1998). *Legal and ethical dilemmas surrounding prayer as a method of alternative healing for children.* Humana Press.

Network for Public Health Law. (2019). *State lead testing policies for children not enrolled in Medicaid: 50-state survey.* https://www.networkforphl.org/wp-content/uploads/2019/12/50-State-Survey-Lead-Screening-for-Children-Not-Enrolled-in-Medicaid.pdf

Noonan, A. S., Velasco-Mondragon, H. E., & Wagner, F. A. (2016). Improving the health of African Americans in the USA: An overdue opportunity for social justice. *Public Health Reviews, 37*(12), 1–20. https://doi.org/10.1186/s40985-016-0025-4

Omer, S. B., Enger, K. S., Moulton, L. H., Halsey, N. A., Stokley, S., & Salmon, D. A. (2008). Geographic clustering of nonmedical exemptions to school immunization requirements and associations with geographic clustering of pertussis. *American Journal of Epidemiology, 168,* 1389–1396.

Ontario Consultants on Religious Tolerance. (n.d.). http//www.religioustolerance.org

Opel, D. J., & Omer, S. B. (2015). Measles, mandates, and making vaccination the default option. *JAMA Pediatrics, 16*(4), 303–304.

Orr, R. (2003). Faith-based decisions: Parents who refuse appropriate care for their children. *Virtual Mentor, 5*(8), 223–225. doi: 10.1001/virtualmentor.2003.5.8.ccas1-0308

Osterberg, L., & Blaschke, T. (2005). Adherence to medication. *New England Journal of Medicine, 353*(5), 487–497.

Overbay, J. D. (1996). Parental participation in treatment decisions for pediatric oncology and intensive care unit patients. *Dimensions of Critical Care Nursing, 15*(1), 16–24.

Panico, M. L., Jenq, G. Y., & Brewster, U. C. (2011). When a patient refuses life-saving care: Issues raised when treating a Jehovah's Witness. *American Journal of Kidney Diseases, 58*(4), 647–653.

Parasidis, E., & Opel, D. J. (2017). Parental refusal of childhood vaccines and medical neglect laws. *American Journal of Public Health, 107*(1), 68–71. https://doi.org/10.2105/AJPH.2016.303500

Paris, J. (1982). Terminating treatment for newborns: A theological perspective. *Law, Medicine and HealthCare, June,* 120–124.

Paris, J., & Bell, A. (1993). Guarantee my child will be "normal" or stop all treatment. *Journal of Perinatology, (13)*6, 469–472.

People v. New York, Peirson. (1903).

Perkin, R., Young, T., Freier, M., Allen, J., & Orr, R. (1997). Stress and distress in pediatric nurses: Lessons from Baby K. *American Journal of Critical Care, 6*(3), 225–232.

Pfuntner, A., Wier, L. M., & Elixhauser, A. (2013). *Overview of hospital stays in the United States, 2011*. HCUP Statistical Brief #166. Agency for Healthcare Research and Quality.

Pierik, R. (2017). On religious and secular exemptions: A case study of childhood vaccination waivers. *Ethnicities, 17*(2), 220–241. https://doi.org/10.1177/1468796817692629

Prager, J., & Rubin, J. (2018). *When a patient refuses treatment, what should doctors do?* https://www.cuimc.columbia.edu/news/when-patient-refuses-treatment-what-should-doctors-do

Prince v. Massachusetts, 321. U.S. 158. (1943–1944).

Purssell, E. (1995). Listening to children: Medical treatment and consent. *Journal of Advanced Nursing, 21*(4), 623–624.

Queensland Health. (2013). *Medicines/pharmaceuticals of animal origin*. Document number QH-GDL-954:2013. https://www.health.qld.gov.au/__data/assets/pdf_file/0024/147507/qh-gdl-954.pdf

Quintero, C. (1993). Blood administration in pediatric Jehovah's Witnesses. *Pediatric Nursing, 19*(1), 46–48.

Radcliffe, S. (2018). When a parent's beliefs about medicine become child abuse. *Healthline*. https://www.healthline.com/health-news/parents-beliefs-about-medicine-child-abuse#1

Reaves, J. (2001, Feb. 1). *Freedom of religion or state-sanctioned child abuse?* http://content.time.com/time/nation/article/0,8599,100175,00.html

Redford, G. (2021, March 2). 6 myths about the COVID-19 vaccines—debunked. *Association of American Medical Colleges*. https://www.aamc.org/news-insights/6-myths-about-covid-19-vaccines-debunked

Reich, J. (2019). Why parents refuse to vaccinate their children, in their own words. *Advisory Board*. https://www.advisory.com/daily-briefing/2019/05/13/antivax

Rhodes, A. (1995). Guardianship and the refusal of treatment. *Maternal Child Nursing*, March/April, 109.

Rhodes, A. M., & Miller, R. D. (1984). *Nursing and the law*. Aspen Systems Corp.

Ringnes, H. K., & Hegstad, H. (2016). Erratum to: Refusal of medical blood transfusions among Jehovah's Witnesses: Emotion regulation of the dissonance of saving and sacrificing life. *Journal of Religion and Health, 56*(1), 370.

Rosaldo, R. (1993). *Culture and truth: The remaking of social analysis* (2nd ed.). Beacon.

Rubak, S., Sandbaek, A., Lauritzen, T., & Christensen, B. (2005). Motivational interviewing: A systematic review and meta-analysis. *British Journal of General Practice, 55*, 305–312.

Rubinkam, M. (2017, Feb. 1). *2-year-old girl dies after faith-healing parents refuse medical treatment: Officials*. https://www.nbcphiladelphia.com/news/national-international/ella-foster-faith-healing-death/29977/

REFERENCES

Ruccione, K., Kramer, R., Moore, I., & Perin, G. (1991). Informed consent for treatment of childhood cancer: Factors affecting parents' decision making. *Journal of Pediatric Oncology Nursing, 8*(30), 112–121.

Rutledge, B. (2011). *Cultural differences - the power distance relationship.* https://thearticulateceo.typepad.com/my-blog/2011/09/cultural-differences-the-power-distance-relationship.html#:~:text=Power%20distance%20refers%20to%20the,do%20peop le%20i

Sattar, S. P., Ahmed, M. S., Madison J., Olsen, D. R., Bhatia, S. C., Ellahi, S., . . . Wilson, D. R. (2004). Patient and physician attitudes to using medications with religiously forbidden ingredients. *Annals of Pharmacotherapy 38*(11), 1830–1835. doi:10.1345/aph.1E001

Scibilia, J. P. (2018). Document "informed refusal" just as you would informed consent. *AAP News.* https://www.aappublications.org/news/2018/10/30/law103018

Selde, W. (2015). Know when and how your patient can legally refuse care. *Journal of Emergency Medical Services, 3*(40). https://www.jems.com/2015/03/25/know-when-and-how-your-patient-can-legal/

Shen, W. (2019). *An overview of state and federal authority to impose vaccination requirements.* Congressional Research Service. https://fas.org/sgp/crs/misc/LSB10300.pdf

Spooner, K., Salemi, J., Salihu, H., & Zoorob, R. (2017). Discharge against medical advice in the United States, 2002–2011. *Mayo Clinic Proceedings, 92*(4), 5–35.

Srinivasan, M., & Pooler, J. (2018). Cost-related medication nonadherence for older adults participating in SNAP. *American Journal of Public Health, 108*(2), 224–230.

Stanhope, M., & Lancaster, J. (2016). *Public health nursing: Population-centered health care in the community* (9th ed.). Elsevier.

Sundin-Huard, D., & Fahy, K. (1999). Moral distress, advocacy and burnout; theorizing the relationships. *International Journal of Nurse Practitioners, 5*(1), 8–13.

Swan, R. (n.d.). *CHILD's public policy achievements.* http://childrenshealthcare.org/?page_id=24

Swan, R. (1997). Children, medicine, religion, and the law. *Advances in Pediatrics, 44*, 491–544.

Swan, R. (2000, November). When faith fails children. *The Humanist, 16*(6).

Swan, R. (2020a). *Churches and movements listed below have religious beliefs against some or most forms of medicine.* http://childrenshealthcare.org/?page_id=195

Swan, R. (2020b). *Victims of religious-based medical neglect.* http://childrenshealthcare.org/?page_id=132

Talbot, N. (1983). The position of the Christian Science Church. *The New England Journal of Medicine, 309*(26), 1641–1644.

Teijaro, J. R., & Farber, D. L. (2021). COVID-19 vaccines: Modes of immune activation and future challenges. *Nature Reviews Immunology, 21,* 195–197. doi: https://doi.org/10.1038/s41577-021-00526-x

Thurkauf, G. (1989). Understanding the beliefs of Jehovah's Witnesses. *Focus on Critical Care, 16*(3), 199–204.

Tierney, W., Weinberger, M., Greene, J., & Studdard, A. (1984). Jehovah's Witnesses and blood transfusion: Physicians' attitudes and legal precedent. *Southern Medical Journal, 77*(4), 473–477.

Torrey, T. (2020). Do patients have the right to refuse medical treatment? *Verywell Health.* www.verywellhealth.com/do-patients-have-the-right-to-refuse-treatment-2614982

University of Virginia, Frank Batten School of Leadership and Public Policy. (2020). *Black Americans are systematically under-treated for pain. Why?* https://batten.virginia.edu/about/news/black-americans-are-systematically-under-treated-pain-why#

Veins, A. M., McGowan, C. R., & Vass, C. M. (2020, June 23). Moral distress among healthcare workers: Ethics support is a crucial part of the puzzle. *BMJ Opinion.* https://blogs.bmj.com/bmj/2020/06/23/moral-distress-among-healthcare-workers-ethics-support-is-a-crucial-part-of-the-puzzle/

Vercillo, A., & Duprey, S. (1988). Jehovah's Witnesses and the transfusion of blood products. *New York State Journal of Medicine, September,* 493–494.

Vermontethicsnetwork.org. (2021). *Right to refuse medical treatment.* www.vtethicsnetwork.org/medical-ethics/right-to-refuse-treatment

Vigo, A., Costagliola, G., Ferrero, E., & Noce, S. (2017). Hypotonic-hyporesponsive episodes after administration of hexavalent DTP-based combination vaccine: A description of 12 cases. *Human Vaccines & Immunotherapeutics, 13*(6), 1375–1378. https://doi.org/10.1080/21645515.2017.1287642

Wang, E., Clymer, J., Davis-Hayes, C., & Buttenheim, A. (2014). Nonmedical exemptions from school immunization requirements: A systematic review. *American Journal of Public Health, 104*(11), e62–e84.

Warraich, H. J. (2009). Religious opposition to polio vaccine. *Emerging Infectious Diseases, 15*(6), 978.

Washington, H. A. (2006). *Medical apartheid: The dark history of medical experimentation on black Americans from colonial times to the present* (1st ed.). Harlem Moon.

Watchko, J. F. (1983). Decision making on critically ill infants by parents. *American Journal of Diseases of Children, 137*(8), 795–798.

Weller, E. R. (2017). Caring for the Amish: What every anesthesiologist should know. *Anesthesia and Analgesia, 124*(5), 1520–1528.

REFERENCES

West Virginia Legislature. (2018). *Senate Bill 337*. https://www.wvlegislature.gov/Bill_Status/bills_text.cfm?billdoc=SB337%20INTR.htm&yr=2018&sesstype=RS&i=337

Whisenant, D. P. (2019). *Power distance in healthcare: Learning from aviation to decrease power distance and improve healthcare culture* [Presentation]. Sigma Theta Tau International Research Congress, Calgary, Alberta, Canada. https://stti.confex.com/stti/congrs19/webprogram/Paper98235.html

Wilkinson, D., & Savulescu, J. (2018). *Ethics, conflict and medical treatment for children: From disagreement to dissensus*. Elsevier. https://www.ncbi.nlm.nih.gov/books/NBK537980/

Wilson, J. (2016, April 13). Letting them die: Parents refuse medical help for children in the name of Christ. *The Guardian*. https://www.theguardian.com/us-news/2016/apr/13/followers-of-christ-idaho-religious-sect-child-mortality-refusing-medical-help

Winiarski, D., Klatt, E., & Kazerouninia, A. (2018). *Risks and legal issues in caring for minor Jehovah's Witness patients*. The American Society for Health Care Risk Management. https://forum.ashrm.org/2018/03/29/risks-and-legal-issues-in-caring-for-minor-jehovahs-witness-patients/

World Health Organization. (2008). *Bulletin of the World Health Organization, Vol. 86*. https://www.who.int/bulletin/volumes/86/en/

World Health Organization. (2020). *DNA vaccines*. https://www.who.int/biologicals/areas/vaccines/dna/en/

INDEX

NOTE: Page references noted with a *t* are tables.

A

AAP Committee on Bioethics, 61
abuse
   child abuse, 66, 67, 75–77, 209–210
   Child Abuse Prevention and Treatment Act of 1974, 73, 74, 77–79, 166
   spiritual abuse, 211–212
acceptable blood-related products (JW), 127*t*–129*t*
actions, legal, 67–70
adjuvants, vaccines, 37
adolescent refusal cases, 68–70. *See also* children
adult healthcare, cultural diversity in, 146
adult refusal, 14–15
   alternative therapies, 102–105
   avoidant health-seeking behaviors, 98–102
   communication, 90–95
   COVID-19, 106, 107–108
   global distrust of vaccines, 108–110
   global perspectives on health, 96–97
   Health Belief Model (HBM), 94–95
   individual worldview, 97–98
   interventions, 88–89
   medication nonadherence, 89–90
   vaccines, 105–108
Adventist Health Study (AHS-2), 117
advocacy, 56
African American males. *See also* Black community; cultures
   avoidant health-seeking behaviors, 98–102
   medication nonadherence, 89
   Tuskegee experiment, 12, 100

allopathic medical treatments, 22–23
  benefits of, 26
  philosophical-based treatment refusals, 24–25
alternative therapies, 102–105, 188
  to blood transfusions, 125t–127t, 133
  prayer as, 119–120
alternative treatments, 11, 115
American Academy of Pediatrics (AAP), 61, 74, 163, 164, 169
American Civil Liberties Union, 79
American Heritage College Dictionary, 61
American Medical Association (AMA), 87, 88, 99
  religious exemptions for vaccines, 137
animal-based insulin, 9
animal-based pharmaceuticals, 147t–148t
antibodies, 34
antigens, 36
anti-science perspectives, 32
anti-vaccination movement, 24. *See also* vaccines
anti-vax parents, 32. *See also* childhood vaccines
anti-vaxxers, 207. *See also* vaccines
assent, 61–62
Asser, Seth, 165
assessments, 171
Associated Jehovah's Witnesses for Reform on Blood (AJWRB), 133
asthma, 36
AstraZeneca, 34
autism, 36
auto-immune diseases, 36
autologous blood, 128t
autonomy, 3, 48, 53, 54, 68
auto-transfusions, 131
avoidant health-seeking behaviors, 98–102

B

Baby Doe regulation, 73, 74
Bates, Amanda, 120
beef-based insulin, 9
behaviors, learned, 174
belief systems, 1, 2, 22. *See also* religion
  See also religious doctrines
  case examples of refusal cases, 176–179, 182–184
  and conduct, 82
  Health Belief Model (HBM), 94–95
  pride in, 180
  treatment refusals, 22–23
beneficence, 53
best interest doctrines, 54
Bible. *See also* religion
  Book of James (King James version), 141
  Followers of Christ Church, 140
  interpretations of, 162
  Jehovah's Witnesses, 122 (*see also* Jehovah's Witnesses)
Bible Reading Fellowship, 113
bipolar disorder, 14
Black community
  avoidant health-seeking behaviors, 98–102
  Tuskegee experiment, 12, 100
blood-based treatments
  acceptable blood-related products (JW), 127t–129t
  Jehovah's Witnesses, 125
blood donations, 129t
blood transfusions, 5–6, 26
  alternatives to, 125t–127t, 133
  and Jehovah's Witnesses, 123, 124 (*see also* Jehovah's Witnesses)
  resources, 214–215
Boise, Idaho, 165

INDEX

books, 216–217. *See also* research; resources
boosters, vaccines, 33. *See also* vaccines
Boulder Weekly, 167, 168
bovine pharmaceutical products, 148*t*
breastfeeding, 40
Brown, Ruth, 142
Byrd, Randolph, 119

C

Canada, 70–71
cancer, 16
    hands-on prayer and, 7–8
capacity, presence of, 66
Caplan, Arthur, 50
capsid, 33
cardiopulmonary bypass technology, 131
case examples, 5
    adult refusal scenarios, 14–15
    alternative treatments, 11
    cultural care, 7
    culture and tradition, 9
    deferred health maintenance, 15–17
    faith and disease, 6
    faith-based refusals, 11
    faith healing, 10
    hands-on prayer, 7–8
    hormone replacement therapy (HRT), 19
    immunization refusals, 19–20
    nondisclosure of deaths, 9–10
    refusing transfusions, 5–6
    shunning medical care, 10
    traditional healers, 8–9
    treatment compromise scenarios, 13–14
    vaccine refusal and cultural perspectives, 12
    vaccine refusal and philosophy, 12–13
    vaccine refusal and religion, 11–12
cells, death of, 40
Centers for Disease Control (CDC), 42, 44, 92
    CDC-INFO Contact Center, 217
    talking points on health literacy, 93–94
child abuse. *See* abuse; children
Child Abuse Prevention and Treatment Act of 1974, 73, 74, 77, 79, 166
childhood vaccines, 3, 31–32. *See also* vaccines
    delay, 36
    hesitancy, 41–42
    laws and exceptions, 42–45
    mandates, 42
    responses to concerns, 34–41
    side-effects of, 38
    types of vaccines, 32–35
children
    abuse, 66, 67, 75–77 (*see also* abuse)
    assent, 61–62
    case examples of refusal cases, 176–179
    children's rights, 48–52
    Christian Scientists and, 136
    common concerns about vaccine administration, 203–205
    consent, 60 (*see also* consent)
    death of, 26, 142, 143
    emancipation, 68
    emotional reactions in refusal cases, 154–159
    ethics, 53–57
    Followers of Christ Church, 140–143
    history of refusal cases, 71–74
    influence of religiosity on healthcare, 115–119
    informed consent, 60–61

and Jehovah's Witnesses, 124, 132
journalist reactions to refusal cases, 165–170
laws protecting well-being of, 66
medical interventions, 48
medical neglect of, 155
mental capabilities of, 189
no code status, 67
parental permission, 62–63
parent rights ethical doctrines, 54
pediatric healthcare, 47–48 (see also pediatric healthcare)
reasons for treatment refusals, 187–189
and refusal cases, 50, 51 (see also refusal cases)
religious doctrines, 111–112 (see also religious doctrines)
of religious objectors, 80–81
religious-based treatment refusals, 22–23
rights, 79
Supreme Court (US), 49, 50
treatment of, 3–5
vaccines (see childhood vaccines)
Children's Act of 1989 (UK), 68
Children's Hospital of Philadelphia, 39
CHILD USA, 26, 76, 80, 83, 142
Chinese medicine, 11
culture-based treatment refusals, 23
Christ Church (Oregon), 114
Christianity, 9, 10. See also religion
children's healthcare frameworks, 112–115
Dutch Protestant-Christian congregations, 12
religious doctrines (see religious doctrines)
Christian Nursing Society, 162

Christian Scientists, 6, 76, 180, 199. See also exemptions (religious)
and children, 136
Medicare/Medicaid, 137
and prayer, 137
religious doctrines, 134–140
churches, 81. See also religion
children's healthcare frameworks, 112–115
doctrines, 81 (see also religious doctrines)
clergy. See also religion
case examples of refusal cases, 179–181
responsibility and laws, 81–83
clerical interpretations, 119–121
faith healing, 120–121
prayer as therapy, 119–120
clinical practice, suggestions for, 156–157
collaboration, 14
College of Physicians of Philadelphia, 12, 23
colloids, 130
Colorado House Bill 1286, 167, 168
comfort care, 48
Committee of Bioethics of the American Academy of Pediatrics (AAP), 51, 163, 164
committees, decision-making, 154
Commonweal Cancer Help Program, 119
communication
adult refusal, 90–95
confusion and, 92–94
cross-cultural interviews, 102
motivational interviewing, 92
negotiations, 4
refusal cases, 1 (see also refusal cases)
vaccine refusal, 109

INDEX

communities
  case examples of refusal cases, 179–181
  disenfranchised, 12
competence, decision-making, 68
complementary and alternative medicine (CAM), 102–105
complementary therapies, prayer as, 119–120
comprehension skills, 28
compromises, treatment scenarios, 13–14
conduct, beliefs and, 82, 83
conflicts
  ethics and, 56
  treatment and needs, 1–3
  vaccines, 1
conjugate vaccines, 33
conscientious objectors, 27, 188
consent, 59, 60, 187, 189
  assent, 61–62
  informed, 60–61
  parental permission, 62–63
  power distance, 172
  procedures, 27
consistency, 153
Constitution (US), 48, 83. *See also* laws; rights
  First Amendment protection, 82, 83
contamination, lead poisoning, 85
costs, 189
costs (financial), 28
Court of Civil Appeals of Oklahoma (2001), 199
court orders, 8–9
COVID-19, 34, 207–208
  hesitancy/refusal of vaccines, 106, 107–108
  moral distress, 158
  safety of vaccines, 41
  vaccines, 207–208
Crawford, Jennifer, 169

cross-cultural interviews, 102
crystalloid intravenous solutions, 130
Cult Education Institute, 141
cultural care, 7
cultural competence, 145–148
  decision-making models, 151–154
  emotional reactions in refusal cases, 154–159
  moral distress, 158–159
  theoretical influences, 149–151
cultural doctrines, refusal cases and, 1, 2
cultural perspectives, vaccine refusal and, 12
cultures
  animal-based pharmaceuticals, 147*t*–148*t*
  avoidant health-seeking behaviors, 98–102
  case examples of refusal cases, 176–184, 182–184
  cross-cultural interviews, 102
  cultural competence (*see* cultural competence)
  definitions of, 145
  healthcare, 145, 146
  Latinx, 96
  learned behaviors and, 174
  studying, 174, 175
  and tradition, 9
  treatment refusals, 23
curandero (traditional native healer), 8

D

deafness, 36
death
  of cells, 40
  of children, 26, 142, 143
  Followers of Christ Church and, 140–143
  nondisclosure of, 9–10

decision-making. *See also* parental decisions
  assumptions, 154
  case examples of refusal cases, 176–184
  competence, 68
  implications of religion on, 124
  models, 150, 151–154
  parental decisions (*see* parental decisions)
  pressures of decisions, 189
  religious doctrines and, 115 (*see also* religious doctrines)
deferred health maintenance, 15–17
DeGeus-Morris, Vicki, 169
delays
  adult refusal, 87–89, 91
  childhood vaccines, 36
  treatments, 27
depression, 14, 15
diabetes, 9, 96
diets, 26, 40
disease detection, 47
disenfranchised communities, 12
disinterest, 152
dispassion, 153
distance, power. *See* power distance
distrust of vaccines, 108–110, 180
diversity in healthcare, 146
DNA vaccines, 33–34
doctrines
  best interest, 54
  church, 81
  ethics, 55 (*see also* ethics)
  legal pertaining to adolescents, 70
  parent rights ethical, 54
  philosophical, 1, 2, 57
  religious, 55, 111–112 (*see also* religious doctrines)
Dominican University of California, 48
Duff, S., 153
Dutch Protestant-Christian congregations, 12
Dyer, Joel, 167, 168

E

Eddy, Mary Baker, 134, 135–136. *See also* Christian Scientists
education
  health, 47
  immunization in public schools, 80
  levels of decision-makers, 28
egalitarianism, modified, 153
Ehrlichman, John, 166
emancipation, 68
emergency department (ED), 8
emotional reactions in refusal cases, 154–159
encephalitis, 38
encephalopathy, 38
Endtime Ministries, 10, 114
enhancers, vaccines, 37
epidemics, 42. *See also* COVID-19; vaccines
epidemiologic studies, 116
epidural blood patches, 129*t*
equine pharmaceutical products, 148*t*
erythropoietin, 130
ethics, 2
  conflicts and, 56
  parent rights ethical doctrines, 54
  pediatric healthcare, 53–57
ethnographic research. *See also* research
  case examples of refusal cases, 176–184
  definitions of, 173–176
evangelical Christians, 10
exemptions (religious), 75–77. *See also* religion
  clergy responsibility and laws, 81–83
  Committee of Bioethics (AAP), 163, 164
  historical influences, 77–81
  treatments, 83–85
  vaccines, 42–45
  for vaccines, 137

INDEX

F

faith, 6. *See also* faith healing; religion
    psychodynamics of, 117
    relationships between health and, 116
    treatment refusals, 22–23
Faith Assembly Church, 11
faith-based refusals, 11
faith healing, 10, 26, 114, 120–121
    Followers of Christ Church, 140–143
Faith Tabernacle Congregation Church, 114, 166
families. *See also* parental decisions
    children and, 3–5 (*see also* children)
    decision-making models, 150, 151–154
    of Jehovah's Witnesses (JW), 155
family nurse practitioner (FNP), 13
fatalism, 100
females, Non-Hispanic Black women, 99
First Amendment protection, 82, 83
Followers of Christ Church, 140–143, 169
food-as-medicine, 97
forced treatments, 155
freedom from nonconsensual invasion, 66
Frost, Norman, 152, 153
fundamentalist Christians, 9, 180

G

General Assembly Church of the Firstborn, 114, 120
global perspectives on health, 96–97
grief, 155
Guardian, 165

guardianship. *See also* parental decisions
    loss of, 26, 57, 197–201
    power distance, 172
    temporary, 66
guidelines
    for children's rights, 49
    Committee of Bioethics (AAP), 164
    staff (for parental refusal), 191–194
guiding principles, 24–25. *see also* philosophy
Guillain-Barre syndrome, 38

H

Haldeman, J.R., 166
hands-on prayer, 7–8
Hayflick limit, 40
healing. *See also* treatment
    belief in God's power, 120
    faith, 10 (*see also* faith healing)
    relationships between health and, 116
    supernatural, 115
health
    avoidant health-seeking behaviors, 98–102
    education, 47
    global perspectives on, 96–97
    literacy, 92, 93–94
    maintenance, 15–17
    relationship between health and, 116
Health Belief Model (HBM), 94–95
healthcare
    cultures, 145, 146
    pediatric, 47–48 (*see also* pediatric healthcare)
heart-lung machine technology, 129t
herd immunity, 24, 40. See also vaccines
heredity, 116

hesitancy, vaccines, 41–42, 90, 105–108, 203–205, 207–208
  COVID-19, 106, 107–108, 207–208
hierarchies, 172. *See also* interventions; parental decisions
Hindus, cultural norms of, 146
Hispanic males, medication nonadherence, 89
history of refusal cases, 71–74
Hofstede, Geert, 182
holistic treatments, 115
hormone replacement therapy (HRT), 19
hospice care, 48
Houseman, Denise, 166
hypertension and religious groups, 117
hypotonic/hyporesponsive episodes, 39

I

Idaho Statesmen, 142
illnesses
  detection, 47
  sudden illness needs, 48
immunity. *See also* vaccines
  herd, 24, 40
  natural, 39
immunization. *See also* childhood vaccines; vaccines
  common concerns, vaccine administration, 203–205
  hesitancy, 90
  for newborns, 78
  in public schools, 80
  refusals, 19–20
  trust in vaccines, 207–208
Immunization Action Coalition (IAC), 217
Indiana Supreme Court, 73

individuality, 12
individual worldview, adult refusal, 97–98
influence, 112, 188. *See also* parental decisions; religious doctrines
  case examples of refusal cases, 182–184
  on children's healthcare, 115–119
  of cultural groups, 146
  professional interventions and, 172 (*see also* professional interventions)
  theoretical, 149–151
information sources
  conflicts, 188
  research, 213–217
informed consent, 60–61
informed refusal, 151
Institute of Noetic Studies, 115
insulin, animal-based, 9
interventions, 48, 88–89
  case examples of refusal cases, 176–184
  courts overriding parental rights, 200–201
  limitations on, 187
  professional, 171–173 (*see also* professional interventions)
interviews, cross-cultural, 102

J

Jacobsen v. Massachusetts (1905), 44, 72
Jarrett, Arthur, 168
Jehovah's Witnesses (JW), 122–134, 180
  acceptability of procedures for, 130
  acceptable blood-related products, 127t–129t
  alternatives to blood transfusions, 125t–127t

INDEX

Associated Jehovah's Witnesses for Reform on Blood (AJWRB), 133
blood-based treatments, 125
blood transfusions and, 123, 124
censure of members, 132
children and, 124, 132
Christian Nursing Society, 162
consequences of disobedience, 123
contracts with physicians and, 132
families of, 155
New World Translation, 122
refusal cases, 132
theoretical influences, 149–150
Jews, cultural norms of, 146
Johnson & Johnson, 34
journalists, reactions to refusal cases, 165–170
judgment, substituted, 54
juries, decision-making, 154
justice, 53

K–L

Koch, Robert, 96
Kostinchuk, David, 168, 169

The Lancet, 36, 37
Larabee, Mark, 140, 168
Latinx cultures, 96
laws
   best interest and, 209–210
   child abuse, 75–77
   Child Abuse Prevention and Treatment Act of 1974, 73, 74, 77, 79
   Children's Act of 1989 (UK), 68
   children's rights, 48–52
   clergy responsibility and, 81–83
   court orders, 8–9
   exemptions (*See* exemptions [religious])
   influence of religious groups, 80
   legal actions, 67–70
   legal perspectives of treatments, 65–67
   loss of guardianship, 197–201
   principles, 2
   protecting well-being of children, 66
   reasons to override refusal, 67–68
   US Constitution, 48, 82
   vaccines, 42–45
laying on hands, 114
lead poisoning, 85
Lerner, Michael, 119
leukocyte transfusions, 131
Levin, Jeffery S., 116, 117
limitations
   adult refusal, 87–89, 91
   emotional reactions in refusal cases, 155
   on interventions, 187
literacy, health, 92, 93–94
live virus vaccines, 32
loss of guardianship, 197–201

M

Macklin, Ruth, 51
maintenance, health, 15–17
males
   African American (*see* African American males)
   medication nonadherence, 89
management
   common concerns about vaccine administration, 203–205
   medication, 90
   staff guidelines (for parental refusal), 191–194
mandates
   childhood vaccines, 42
   vaccines, 24

Massachusetts Supreme Judicial Court, 67
mature minors, 70. See also adolescents
measles, mumps, rubella (MMR), and varicella vaccines, 32, 38, 39
medical interventions, 48
medical treatment, 1–3
    adolescent refusals, 68–70
    children and families, 3–5
    loss of guardianship, 197–201
    postponement of, 156
    refusal cases, 1
    shunning, 10
Medicare FFS [fee-for-service] expenditures, 89
Medicare/Medicaid, Christian Scientists, 137
medication
    alternative therapies, 102–105
    animal-based pharmaceuticals, 147t–148t
    food-as-medicine, 97
    management, 90
    nonadherence, 89–90
    vaccines (see vaccines)
mental capacity of parents, 189
mercury, 37
messenger RNA (mRNA) vaccines, 34
metabolic testing for newborns, 78
Mexico, culture-based treatment refusals, 23
Miller, William R., 90
minors, 26. See also children
mistrust, 180
mobile device apps, 216
models
    decision-making, 150, 151–154
    Health Belief Model (HBM), 94–95
Moderna, 34
modified egalitarianism, 153
moral distress, 158–159, 178
    common concerns, vaccine administration, 203–205
    trust in vaccines, 207–208
Moral Distress Scale, 159
moral force, concept of, 156
morbidity, 116
mortality rates, 99, 116
motivation, Health Belief Model (HBM), 94–95
motivational interviewing, 91, 92
murine pharmaceutical products, 148t
Muslims, 7, 9
    cultural norms of, 146
    culture-based treatment refusals, 23

N

National Cancer Institute, 61
National Center for Health Statistics (NCHS), 102–105. See also alternative therapies
National Health Interview Survey (2013-2015), 90
Native Americans, culture-based treatment refusals, 23
natural immunity, 39. See also vaccines
needs, patient. See patient needs
negotiations, 171
    refusal cases, 4
newborns. See also children
    immunization for, 78
    metabolic testing for, 78
The New England Journal of Medicine, 138
Newmark v. Williams (1991), 199
New World Translation, 122
New York State Psychiatric Institute, 100
The New York Times, 100

INDEX

New York University, 50
Nixon, Richard M., 166
no, reasons for saying, 92–94. *See also* adult refusal; refusal cases
no code status, 67
nondisclosure
 of alternative medicine, 103
 of deaths, 9–10
non-maleficence, 53
nursing
 advocacy, 56
 reactions to refusal cases, 162–163
 staff guidelines (for parental refusal), 191–194
 stress of, 156

O

Office of the United Nations High Commissioner for Human Rights, 49
Ohio State University, 50
omnipercipience, 152
omniscience, 152
The Oregonian, 140, 168

P

packed red blood cell transfusions, 131
palliative care, 48
pandemics, 34, 207–208
parental decisions, 51
 assent, 61–62
 case examples of refusal cases, 176–181
 for children, 3
 children's rights and, 48–52
 decision-making models, 150, 151–154
 exemptions, 75–77 (*see also* exemptions [religious])
 history of refusal cases, 71–74
 informed consent, 60–61 (*see also* consent)
 loss of guardianship, 197–201
 mental capacity of parents, 28, 189
 parental permission, 62–63
 parent rights ethical doctrines, 54
 power distance, 172
 reasons to override refusal, 67–68
 refusal cases, 66 (*see also* refusal cases)
 relationships, 28, 188
 religious-based treatment refusals, 22–23
 states' rights, 54
 theoretical influences, 149–151
 time frames, 27
 treatment refusal reasons, 26, 187–189
 vaccines, 31–32 (*see also* childhood vaccines)
Pasteur, Louis, 96
pathogens, 39
patient needs, 1–3
 children and families, 3–5
pediatric healthcare, 47–48. *See also* children
 children's rights, 48–52
 cultural diversity in, 146
 ethics, 53–57
Pediatric Society (Canada), Bioethics Committee, 70–71
Pellechia, James, 132
Pentecostal sects, 114
People v. New York, Peirson (1903), 72
perceptions of being right, concept of, 156
perfluorochemicals, 130
permission, 60, 62–63. *See also* consent
Pfizer-BioNTech, 34
pharmaceuticals, animal-based, 147t–148t

philosophical doctrines, 1, 2, 57
philosophy
  treatment refusals, 24–25
  vaccine refusal and, 12–13
phone numbers, 217. *See also* resources
physicians, reactions to refusal cases, 163–165
pig tissue, religion and, 7
plasma proteins, 128*t*
plasma transfusions, 131
platform-based vaccines, 33
poison, lead poisoning, 85
policies, informed consent, 61
polysaccharide conjugate vaccines, 33
porcine pharmaceutical products, 147*t*
pork-based insulin, 9
postoperative cell salvage/reinfusion, 131
postponement of medical treatment, 156
power distance, 171
  case examples of refusal cases, 182–184
Power Distance Index (PDI), 172
practice guidelines, refusal cases, 3
practices, 83. *See also* conduct, beliefs and
prayer, 7–8, 180. *See also* religion
  belief in power of, 114
  Child Abuse Prevention and Treatment Act of 1974, 73, 74
  Christian Scientists and, 137
  efficacy of, 118
  influence on children's healthcare, 115–119
  preference for, 187
  reasons for treatment refusal, 26
  relationship between health and, 116
  religious-based treatment refusals and, 22–23
  research on, 118
  therapeutic effects of, 119–120
  as therapy, 119–120
pregnancy, mortality rates, 99
preoperative cell salvage/reinfusion, 131
preservatives, 37
pressures of decisions, 189
preventative treatments, 83
  of childhood disease, 40
  vaccines, 3 (*see also* childhood vaccines; treatment; vaccines)
Prince v. Massachusetts (1944), 50, 712
principles, guiding, 24–25. *See also* philosophy
privacy, 66. *See also* rights
professional groups
  journalist reaction to refusal cases, 165–170
  nursing reaction to refusal cases, 162–163
  physician reaction to refusal cases, 163–165
  refusal case reactions, 161–162
professional interventions, 171–173
  case examples of refusal cases, 176–184
  research (refusal cases), 173–176
protection, 43. *See also* vaccines
psychodynamics of faith, 117
public schools, immunization in, 79–80

R

recombinant vaccines, 33
refusal cases, 1
  adolescents, 68–69, 70
  adult refusal, 14–15, 87–89 (*see also* adult refusal)
  case examples of, 5, 176–184 (*see also* case examples)
  children and, 50, 51

INDEX

consent (*see* consent)
COVID-19, 105–108
distrust of vaccines, 108–110
emotional reactions in, 154–159
exemptions, 75–77 (*see also* exemptions [religious])
faith-based refusals, 11
history of, 71–74
immunization refusals, 19–20
informed refusal, 151
Jehovah's Witnesses, 132 (*see also* Jehovah's Witnesses [JW])
journalist reactions to, 165–170
loss of guardianship, 197–201
of medical treatment, 156
negotiations, 4
nursing reactions to, 162–163
physician reactions to, 163–165
practice guidelines, 3
professional interventions, 171–173 (*see also* professional interventions)
reactions, 161–162
reasons for treatment refusals, 21, 187–189 (*see also* treatment refusals)
reasons to override, 67–68
religion, 75–77 (*see also* religion)
research, 173–176
rights of adults, 51, 65, 66
vaccine refusal and cultural perspectives, 12
vaccine refusal and philosophy, 12–13
vaccine refusal and religion, 11–12
vaccines, 3
relationships, parental decisions, 28, 188
religion, 75–77
in the Black community, 100
blood transfusions and, 5–6
case examples of refusal cases, 176–179, 182–184

Christian Science practitioners, 6
clergy responsibility and laws, 81–83
consent, 60 (*see also* consent)
doctrines (*see* religious doctrines)
Dutch Protestant-Christian congregations, 12
Endtime Ministries, 10
evangelical Christians, 10
faith and disease, 6
Faith Assembly Church, 11
fundamentalist Christians, 9
hands-on prayer, 7–8
influence of background, 115
Muslims, 7, 9
reasons for treatment refusal, 26
refusal cases and, 1, 2
treatment refusals, 22–23
vaccine refusal and, 11–12
religiosity, influence on children's healthcare, 115–119
religious doctrines, 111–112, 180
children's healthcare frameworks, 112–115
Christian Scientists, 134–140 (*see also* Christian Scientists)
clerical interpretations, 119–121
definitions of, 121–122
Followers of Christ Church, 140–143
influence on children's healthcare, 115–119
Jehovah's Witnesses, 122–134
violations of, 155
religious exemptions. *See* exemptions
religious groups
hypertension and, 117
influence of, 80
research
case examples of refusal cases, 176–184
information sources, 213–217
on prayer, 118
refusal cases, 173–176

249

resistance, 40. *See also* immunity; vaccines
resources
  blood transfusions, 214–215
  mobile device apps, 216
  vaccines, 215–216
rights. *See also* laws
  of adults to refuse treatments, 51, 65, 66
  children, 48–52, 79 (*see also* pediatric healthcare)
  informed consent, 61 (*see also* consent)
  legal actions, 67–70
  loss of guardianship, 197–201
  parent rights ethical doctrines, 54
  privacy, 66 (*see also* privacy)
  self-protection of, 12
  states, 54
  Supreme Court (US), 49, 50
  United Nations Committee on the Rights of the Child, 49
risk factors, 15
Rollnick, Stephen, 90
Rubinkam, Michael, 166
Russell, Charles Taze, 122

S

safety of vaccines, 37–38, 41, 43, 171
salutary effects, 116
Science and Health, With Key to the Scripture (Eddy), 134
screenings, 47, 48
secular beliefs, 83
secular conduct, 83
seizures, 36
self-determination, 50
self-protection of rights, 12
shaman, 8
shunning medical care, 10
side-effects of vaccines, 38
Simms, Marion J., 99

skin grafts, 7
smallpox, 43
SNAP (state nutrition assistance programs), 90
Society of Pediatric Nurses, 169
spike proteins, 34
spiritual abuse, 211–212
spirituality, 22
  religion (*see* religion)
  treatment refusals, 22–23
states
  child abuse, 209–210
  religious exemptions, 75–77, 84*t*–85*t* (*see also* exemptions [religious])
  rights, 54
status, decision-maker, 151. *See also* decision-making; parental decisions
statutes (states), child abuse, 209–210
stem cell transfusions, 128*t*
substituted judgment, 54
subunit vaccines, 33
supernatural healing, 115
support, refusal cases and, 1, 2
Supreme Court (Indiana), 73
Supreme Court (US), 49, 50. *See also* laws; rights
Swift, Gayle, 116
syphilis, 12

T

technology, fear of, 27
temporary guardianship, 66
theoretical influences, 149–151
therapeutic effects of prayer, 119–120
thimerosal, 37
thrombopoietin mimetics, 130
time frames, parental decisions, 27
Time magazine, 165
toxoid vaccines, 33
tradition, culture and, 9
traditional healers, 8–9

INDEX

tranexamic acid (antifibrinolytic), 130
transfusions
    auto-transfusions, 131
    blood, 26 (*see also* blood transfusions)
    Jehovah's Witnesses (*see* Jehovah's Witnesses)
    packed red blood cell, 131
    plasma, 131
    refusing, 5–6
    stem cell, 128*t*
    white blood cell, 128*t*
    whole blood, 130
treatment refusals, 90. *See also* treatments
    adults, 87–89 (*see also* adult refusal)
    case examples of refusal cases, 176–184
    culture, 23
    philosophy, 24–25
    professional interventions, 171–173
    reasons for, 21, 25–29, 187–189
    religion, 22–23
    websites, 214
treatments
    adolescent refusals, 68–70
    alternative, 11, 115
    compromise scenarios, 13–14
    costs, 28
    definition of, 65
    delays, 27
    exemptions (religious), 83–85
    forced, 155
    history of refusal cases, 71–74
    holistic, 115
    legal perspectives of, 65–67
    loss of guardianship, 197–201
    medical, 1–3 (*see also* medical treatment)
    parental decisions (*see* parental decisions)
    preventative, 83
    reasons to override refusal, 67–68
    rights of adults to refuse, 51, 65, 66
    shunning medical care, 10
    syphilis, 12
    vaccines, 3
trust, 180, 207–208
Tuskegee experiment, 12, 100
types of vaccines, 32–35

U

United Kingdom (UK), Children's Act of 1989, 68
United Nations Committee on the Rights of the Child, 49
United States
    food-as-medicine, 97
    religious exemptions, 75–77 (*see also* exemptions [religious]; states)
universal health literacy precautions, 94
University of California, San Francisco, 180
US Constitution, 48, 82. *See also* laws; rights
    First Amendment protection, 82, 83
US Department of Health, Education, and Welfare, 73
US Department of Health and Human Services (DHHS), 73, 79

V

vaccine-preventable diseases (VPDs), 42, 43
vaccines, 1
    adult refusal, 105–108
    breastfeeding, 40
    childhood, 31–32 (*see also* childhood vaccines)

children and, 3
common concerns about administration, 203–205
COVID-19, 106, 107–108, 207–208
cultural perspectives refusal and, 12
culture-based treatment refusals, 23
distrust of, 108–110
hesitancy, 41–42
laws and exemptions, 42–45
mandates, 24
philosophical-based treatment refusals, 24–25
philosophy refusal and, 12–13
refusal and cultural perspectives, 12
religion and refusal, 11–12
religious exemptions for, 137
safety of, 37–38, 41, 43
side-effects of, 38
smallpox, 43
trust in, 207–208
types of, 32–35
Van Biema, David, 165
videos, 217. *See also* resources
viralism, 149
vitamins, 102, 103

W

Watchko, Jon, 152, 153
Watchtower Bible and Tract Society, 122. *See also* Jehovah's Witnesses
Watergate scandal (1974), 166
well-child care, 47. *See also* pediatric healthcare
Western medical treatment refusal, 4, 25. *See also* refusal cases; treatment; treatment refusals
Western medicine, 182, 183
white blood cell transfusions, 128t
whole blood, 127t
transfusions, 130
whole vaccines, 33
witnesses for permissions, 62
women, hormone replacement therapy (HRT), 19
World Health Organization (WHO), 33, 43
Worldwide Church of God, 9

Z

Zucht v. King (1922), 44

www.ingramcontent.com/pod-product-compliance
Lightning Source LLC
Chambersburg PA
CBHW070757230426
43665CB00017B/2390